BSAVA
MANUAL OF ORNAMENTAL FISH

Edited by

_oan Bo

Ray L Butcher
MA VetMB MRCVS

Published by the
British Small Animal
Veterinary Association,
Kingsley House, Church Lane,
Shurdington, Cheltenham,
Gloucestershire GL51 5TQ.

Printed by J. Looker Printers,
Poole, Dorset.

The publishers cannot take any responsibility
for information provided on dosages and methods
of application of drugs mentioned in this publication.
Details of this kind must be verified by individual users
in the appropriate literature.

First published 1992

ISBN 0 905214 18 8

CONTENTS

CONTENTS

ACKNOWLEDGEMENTS

I would like to express my sincere appreciation to all the contributors of this latest manual, not only for the work involved in writing their own chapters, but also for their enthusiasm, patience, and help throughout.

In addition I am indebted to Professor J.B. Gratzek of the University of Georgia, USA for kindly supplying two of the colour photographs.

Matthew Poulson and the staff of J. Looker Printers have given invaluable help and advice with regard to layout and production. Much needed secretarial assistance was provided by Mrs. Penny Bredemear and Mrs. Brenda Burland, and Mr. Andrew Hoey showed extreme patience in helping to develop my word-processing skills.

Both Mr. Harvey Locke and Mr. Simon Orr have been the chairman of the B.S.A.V.A. Publications Committee during the production of this manual, and I am indebted to them for their support.

Lastly, I would like to acknowledge all the encouragement given by fellow B.S.A.V.A. officers, colleagues in my practice, and especially my family, without which the task would have seemed impossible.

CONTRIBUTORS

CHRIS ANDREWS, B.Sc., PhD.
National Aquarium in Baltimore,
Pier 3, 501 East Pratt Street,
Baltimore MD 21202, U.S.A.
Formally: Curator of Aquarium, Invertebrates and
Reptiles, The Zoological Society of London,
Regent's Park, London.

EDWARD J. BRANSON, B.Sc., BVetMed., M.Sc., M.R.C.V.S.
Garden Cottage, Eastnor, Ledbury, Herefordshire. HR8 1RL
Formally: Institute of Aquaculture,
University of Stirling, Stirling, Scotland. FK9 4LA

LYDIA A. BROWN, PhD.,BVSc.,F.R.C.V.S.
Mill Leat, West Gomeldon,
Salisbury, Wilts. SP4 6JZ

RAY L. BUTCHER, M.A., Vet M.B., M.R.C.V.S.
Wylie and Partners,
196 Hall Lane, Upminster, Essex. RM14 1TD

DAVID M. FORD, C.Chem., M.R.S.C., A.I.F.S.T., M.Phil,PhD.
Aquarian Advisory Service,
P.O. Box 67, Elland, West Yorkshire HX5 OS.

PETER J. MILLER, B.Sc., PhD.
Dept. of Zoology, University of Bristol,
Woodland Road, Bristol. BS8 1UG

PETER W. SCOTT, MSc., BVSc., M.R.C.V.S., M.I.Biol.
Keanter, Stoke Charity Road, Kings Worthy,
Winchester, Hants. SO23 7LS

PETER J. SOUTHGATE, BVetMed, MSc., M.R.C.V.S.
2, Manor Farm Cottages, Manor Loan,
Blairlogie, Stirling. FK8 5QA
Formally: Institute of Aquaculture,
University of Stirling, Stirling, Scotland. FK9 4LA

FOREWORD

THE MANUAL OF ORNAMENTAL FISH

The Manual of Ornamental Fish has been produced in response to the rapid growth in importance of this previously neglected field of veterinary medicine. The contents reflect the advances that have been made in our understanding of ornamental fish management and disease and are presented in a practical, easy to use way that is the hallmark of the BSAVA Manual Series.

Ray Butcher has assembled a team of authors, all experts in their field, to contribute to this Manual. The information is presented in a practical and logical way to help the veterinarian in practice understand the important aspects of fish biology and fish keeping, the diseases to which ornamental fish are susceptible, the diagnostic approach to adopt when faced with a problem and the treatment of various diseases. Ray is also to be commended for providing the artwork for all the illustrations.

On behalf of the BSAVA, I would like to thank all the authors for their contributions to this Manual. Particular thanks are due to Ray Butcher for editing the book and to Simon Orr and Harvey Locke, who as successive Chairmen of BSAVA Publications Committee have nurtured and supported the project.

Michael E. Herrtage MA BVSc DVR DVD MRCVS
President, BSAVA

INTRODUCTION

The diagnosis and treatment of diseases of ornamental fish poses the Veterinarian in practice some problems that are distinct from those of treating the more familiar companion animals. Fish are adapted to live in an aquatic environment, and so their anatomy and physiology show variations to those of air-breathing animals. They are in equilibrium with their environment, and with the other organisms within that environment, and any imbalance will predispose to disease. The provision of the correct and stable environment is therefore essential for successful fishkeeping, and the Veterinarian must become familiar with the various methods of monitoring water quality parameters, as well as the wealth of equipment that aquarists have developed to achieve their aims.

A less obvious problem is that the aquarist will often regard his fish as individual companion animals, whereas the disease problem might perhaps more closely resemble that of an intensive livestock situation. Although a great deal of information can be gained from the clinical examination of living fish, specific diagnoses often require post-mortem and laboratory techniques. The aquarist may be unwilling to sacrifice a representative sample of fish for such examinations to be performed.

This manual has been written for the practitioner with these problems in mind. The first section attempts to explain those aspects of fish biology, and fishkeeping in general, that are essential background information to any study of fish diseases. It is also hoped that this section will help the Veterinarian to understand some of the terminology commonly used by aquarists.

Section II is devoted to the different diseases of ornamental fish. For the sake of convenience, each chapter deals with a different category of causative agent, but within that framework the authors have attempted to develop a problem - orientated approach.

Section III outlines the approach a practitioner should adopt when faced with a fish disease problem. No attempt has been made to cover the very important specialist field of histopathology, and the reader is advised to consult the recommended reading list for further information.

The subject of therapeutics is covered in Section IV. This has posed some problems since the current review into the licensing of drugs used in the U.K. may prohibit the future use of some medicaments that are at present commonly available. It is not possible to predict the eventual outcome, and so the information given in this section can only reflect the situation at the time of writing. This same caveat applies to the chapter on legislation.

The appendices are intended to provide a useful, quick reference summary for some of the wealth of information given throughout the rest of the manual.

Ray L. Butcher

CHAPTER ONE

ANATOMY & PHYSIOLOGY

Peter J Miller _____

CLASSIFICATION

Ornamental fish belong almost entirely to the dominant group of living bony fishes named the Teleosts, and, unless otherwise stated, the rest of the chapter refers to this group. Teleosts comprise about 20,000 recent species, showing a wide range of specialisation for different modes of life, in a variety of habitats. Their classification is complex, and the reader is referred to standard texts for details.

Very broadly, the teleosts can be divided into two structural grades :

1. The lower teleosts (more generalised plan, with fusiform bodies, soft fin rays but no conspicuous spiny rays, pectoral fins low on the side of the body, pelvic fins set well back on the abdomen, physostomous swimbladder, and cycloid scales).

2. The higher, spiny-rayed teleosts (with deeper bodies, pectoral fins higher up the sides and pelvics set forward below the pectorals, a physoclistous swimbladder and ctenoid scales).

The lower teleosts comprise fishes such as the salmonids, the carps (with a variety of relatives from tetras and piranhas to loach and catfish), and the eels. The higher teleosts include the perches, sticklebacks, cichlids, gobies, blennies, mackerels and flatfish, and most coral fishes. In between these two major levels, the toothed carps are well represented in aquaria by the killifishes and the poeciliid livebearers, such as guppies and mollies.

A number of teleost groups have been subjected to artificial selection. The results may be seen in the variations in colour, finnage, and head excrescences in goldfish, and the range of vivid colours in Koi carp. More recently, colour and finnage variants have been bred in other smaller aquarium species, such as the barbs, various poeciliid livebearers, like male guppies, swordtails, and platies, as well as the cichlid angel fish and discus. Siamese fighters with flowing fins and red, purple and blue coloration are also the product of domestication.

Other than teleosts, fishes encountered as aquarium species may include the more generalised bony fish, such as the bichir, *Polypterus*, and the North American garfish *Lepisosteus*.

Cartilaginous fishes, including small dogfish and sharks, and the South American freshwater rays, can be recognised by the series of gill slits along the side or underside of the head, and by the upturned or whiplike tail respectively.

EXTERNAL FEATURES

Teleosts vary greatly in body form as an adaptation to their individual habitats and behaviour. The general external features are shown in Fig.1.

FIG. 1: General External Features

Lower teleost pattern (eg. carp).

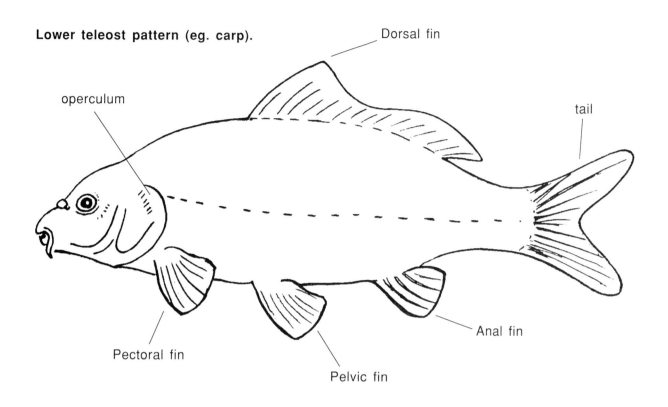

operculum

Dorsal fin

tail

Pectoral fin

Pelvic fin

Anal fin

Higher teleost pattern (eg. perch).

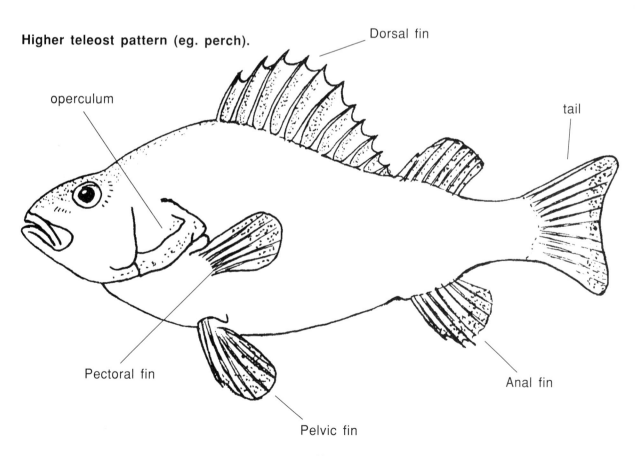

operculum

Dorsal fin

tail

Pectoral fin

Pelvic fin

Anal fin

SKIN

Basic Structure

The structure of the teleost skin is shown in Fig. 2.

The outer part, the epidermis, has several layers of fibrous Malpighian cells, all of which remain living and capable of division despite progressive flattening and fibrous accumulation towards the body surface. The epidermis also houses mucus-secreting goblet cells (which produce glycoproteins), larger clear club cells, and other types, such as granular cells, lymphocytes and macrophages. The epidermis rests on a basement membrane, which separates it from the underlying dermis. The latter contains connective tissue. Below the dermis is a looser, more vascularised and fatty layer, the hypodermis, which separates the skin from the underlying muscle and the skeletal elements of the body.

FIG. 2:
A diagrammatic section through the skin
[Adapted from: *Ichthyology* by Lagler, Bardach, Miller and Passino]

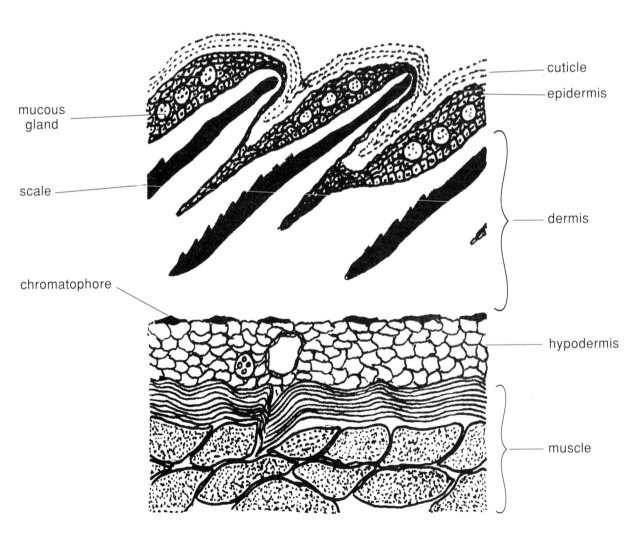

The Cuticle and Mucus

The outermost covering of the epidermis, the cuticle, is a thin mucopolysaccharide layer of cellular material, sloughed cells and mucus. Fish slime, or mucus, is a vital component of the skin/water interface, and is termed the "glycocalyx". It improves locomotion, by reducing frictional drag, and mucus lost from the skin of members of a shoal may affect flow properties of water over the surfaces of other fishes in the shoal.

Mucus also serves a fungicidal and bactericidal function. Damage to mucus cover may contribute to infection of the skin. The layer also has diminished permeability to water, and so aids osmoregulation. In some species mucus is toxic for predators. Among cichlid fishes, some discus (*Symphysodon*) have mucophagous young which feed on skin secretions of the parents. Injured skin in characins and cyprinids releases an alarm pheromone ("Schreckstoff") from the club cells of the epidermis. This induces a flight reaction among the rest of a conspecific group.

Scales

Fish skin typically contains scales, as small dermal skeletal elements, overlapping like roof tiles. In the lower teleosts, these are simple flexible bony plates (cycloid scales), but in more advanced groups, a series of tiny spines (ctenii) is present around the free rear edge of the scale.

Scales originate in scale pockets, and growth around the embedded edge produces a series of fine concentric ridges on the scale surface. The oldest part of the scale is the small focus near the rear apex. Replacement scales regenerated after original scale loss, lack this structure. Spacing of the growth ridges(circulii), and sometimes lines of resorption of mineral material from the growing edge, imprint on the scale an age and growth history of the fish. Under conditions of food shortage or diversion to reproduction, the scale growing edge may be eroded. Some teleosts (eg. eels) have vestigial scales, while others have lost them altogether (such as bullheads).

Coloration

Coloration is determined by pigment or physical effects on skin structure. Pigment is deposited in special cells (chromatophores), which can be black (melanophores) or contain soluble coloured pigments (lipophores). The latter may be either red and orange (erythrophores) or yellow (xanthophores). In the branched melanophores, granules of the black pigment melanin can move within the cell to aggregate (pale), or disperse (darken) under nervous and hormonal influence. The pigments of the lipophores, chiefly carotenoids, come from the food of the fish. Iridocytes contain tiny plates of guanin, a reflecting substance, which produces white, silvery and iridescent effects.

Distinctive colour patterns have evolved for different modes of life and are more or less individually adaptable. Coloration plays a part in concealment, for both prey and predators, by such devices as countershading, dazzle-patterns, eye-spots, background matching, mimicry, or warning. Coloration may also be a means of communication between members of the same species, as in shoaling or in reproductive behaviour (display, courtship, brood control).

LOCOMOTION

Fish movement through the relatively dense medium of water is normally the function of the axial musculature on each side of the body and forming the 'fillet'. The segmented voluntary myotomes are arranged above (epaxial) and below (hypaxial) the lateral midline, inserting on connective tissue attaching to the vertebral column and skin.

Musculature

Axial muscle contains two main sorts of fibre. Most fibres are "white", which contract rapidly for burst swimming, but have little stamina and soon accumulate an oxygen debt. The less numerous "red" fibres contract more slowly, but are highly vascularised and so can sustain activity for longer periods of cruising rather than sprinting. They have a different nerve supply and the proportion of red and white fibres varies with the species' swimming habits. A third, intermediate "pink" fibre occurs in carp and salmonids.

The mechanics of swimming

During swimming, the myotomes contract successively from the anterior end of the body rear-wards, and alternately on each side. This produces waves of lateral bending, pushing the fish forward by a sculling effect. Wave amplitude increases towards the tail and the caudal fin is the final propulsive surface, often displaying more obvious side-to-side motion than the body. In fish of a generalised shape, the caudal fin provides much of the thrust. Typically, larger fish need fewer tail beats to attain a particular speed.

There is a significant reduction of swimming efficiency in water owing to forces from friction and vortex formation. The nature of the skin surface reduces friction, and vortex drag at moderate speeds is minimised by the spindle shaped body, with maximum cross sectional area at about a third or more from the anterior end, tapering towards the tail. The shape of the caudal fin also affects vortex drag, a forked or sickle-shaped fin being most efficient.

Manoeuvrability and Stability

The fins are responsible for manoeuvrability and stability. When extended, all fins can limit rolling, the median fins yawing (swinging from side to side), and the paired fins pitching (vertical dipping and rearing).

In the higher teleosts, such as the perches, the deeper body, the forward shift of the pelvic fins to below the pectorals, and the lateral pectorals, all combine to enhance manoeuvrability. The greater tendency for rolling in the shorter, deeper fish is overcome by having median fins of larger area. The longer-bodied species, such as pike, are stabilised, like an arrow, by more posterior and smaller median fins. The various types of body shape, the distribution and shape of the fins, as well as the proportion of white/red muscle, reflects the many different ways of life for which fish are adapted.

DIGESTION

Teeth usually occur on at least the premaxilla and dentary bones of the jaws. Jaw teeth are absent in cyprinids, which have large pharyngeal teeth biting upwards against a horny pad in the roof of the pharynx.

Much feeding depends on suction caused by the protrusion of the jaws. There are no salivary glands, but the muscular gullet has a folded mucus-secreting lining. Gill-rakers lining the inner edges of the gill arches prevent food loss and assist the active retention of smaller particles from the respiratory water current through the gills. Generally, there is a discrete stomach commencing behind the short gullet, delimited from the intestine by a muscular pyloric sphincter. Often, there is a blind rearward extension of the stomach. In some grazers, like carp, there is no true stomach, while the grey mullet has a muscular gizzard. At the start of the intestine, blind tubular outpushings may be present. These pyloric caecae range from one or a few (perch) to over a hundred (salmonids), and probably enhance enzymic secretion. Gut length is relatively greater in herbivores. The pancreas and gall bladder are normally evident, although the pancreas is variable in appearance. The liver is large and lobulated, and is reddish-brown in colour, although paler in herbivores and cultivated fish.

The digestive enzymes, and the gut pH, are essentially as in higher vertebrates. In carnivores (e.g. trout), most of the stomach is evacuated after about 20 hours , but this varies with the temperature and the meal size, as well as the texture of the food and the size of the fish. In the trout, the assimilation of food is normally about 80% efficient, although at low temperatures less food is eaten and this is assimilated less completely. Food storage, chiefly as triglyceride lipids, can involve much of the body, but typically is concentrated in the liver. The latter becomes large and laden with lipids and glycogen, used for overwintering in temperate conditions, or for fueling reproduction. The processes of digestion, assimilation and deamination of absorbed aminoacids require energy (specific dynamic action), and, in conditions of poor oxygenation, overeating may be fatal.

A diagram of the abdominal viscera is shown in Fig. 3.

FIG.3: A diagram of the abdominal organs

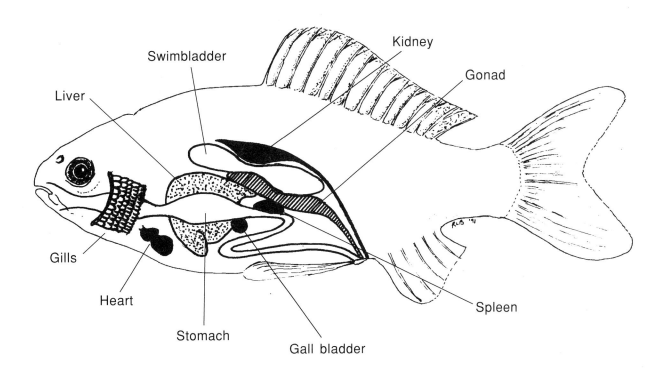

VASCULAR SYSTEM

Teleosts have a single blood circulation, passing only once through the heart, and then to the systemic system directly from the gills. A diagram of the circulation is shown in Fig.4, and of the heart in Fig.5.

Mechanics of Circulation

In trout, the ventricular systolic pressure may range from 30 - 80 mm Hg, and the diastolic values are usually below 30mm Hg. The rate of beating may be as low as 15 / min at 5°C, but rising to about 100 / min at 15°C. The circulation is also helped by body muscular activity and gill contractions, as well as by an elastic ligament along the dorsal aorta in salmonids.

Lymph and Haemopoietic tissue

There is an extensive lymphatic system, containing about four times the blood volume. The capillary walls are very permeable and the lymph closely resembles plasma in its composition. The circulation is helped by lymph "hearts" on the major vessels, and the system supplies the white muscle, which lacks capillaries. The blood volume is relatively low (typically about 5% of body weight). There are no lymph nodes, the chief haemopoietic tissue occurring in the kidney and spleen, where characteristic melanomacrophage centres are formed in conjunction with the white cell system.

FIG 4: The circulation
[Adapted from: *Ichthyology* by Lagler, Bardach, Miller and Passino]

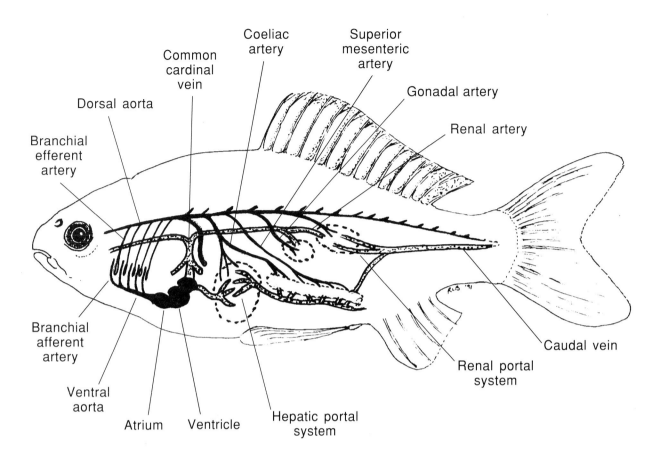

FIG 5: The Heart
[Adapted from: *Ichthyology* by Lagler, Bardach, Miller and Passino]

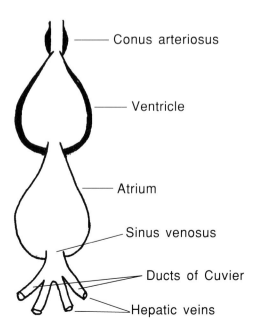

Blood Cells

Erythrocytes are large (typically 12-14 x 8.5-9.5 microns) and nucleated. They metabolise chiefly by oxidative phosphorulation. White cells form up to 10% of the blood cell population, with lymphocytes by far the most abundant, and neutrophils, basophils and monocytes much less frequent than in mammals.

RESPIRATION

Gill Structure

Respiration is based on a system of gills, involving five close-set lateral slits in the pharyngeal wall, with highly vascularised gill filaments supported by skeletal gill arches. The filaments extend from the outer edge of each arch into an opercular chamber which empties to the exterior through a single opening around the edge of the gill-cover. As well as the typical gills, the pseudobranch is a half gill in the upper anterior corner of the opercular chamber (see: Endocrine organs).

The primary lamellae contain skeletal and muscular tissue to permit change of alignment to meet those of the opposite hemibranch. Contact between adjoining arches and between the adjacent lamellae of each arch, produces a fine mesh through which water must pass (Figs.6 and 7). The tiny secondary lamellae form the exchange surface. A counter current system maximises oxygen uptake, which can reach 80%.

FIG. 6 : Structure of the gills

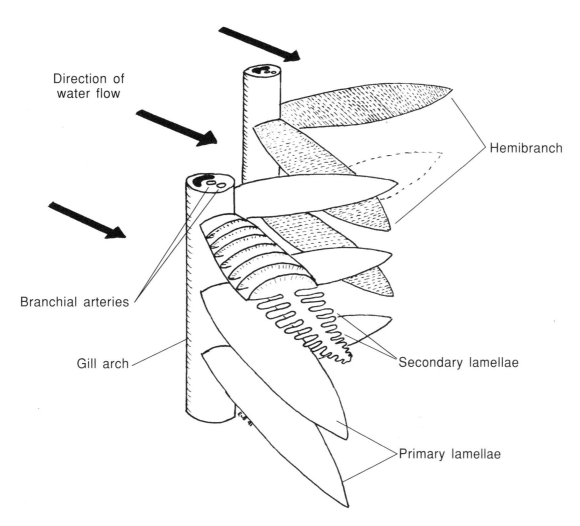

Direction of water flow

Hemibranch

Branchial arteries

Gill arch

Secondary lamellae

Primary lamellae

FIG.7:
The microscopic appearance of the gill lamellae

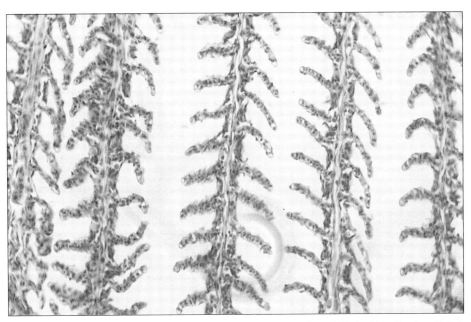

Photo: Ray Butcher   Stained with Haematoxylin and Eosin, Magnification: X 180

Haemoglobins and Oxygen Uptake

Haemoglobins show differences between species in relation to habitat. A Bohr effect is very evident in fish of well oxygenated waters, and an extreme form of this, the Root shift, is peculiar to teleost haemoglobins, when a low pH causes the total oxygen carrying capacity to diminish and influences the shape of the haemoglobin dissociation curve. A high environmental CO_2 level can thus impair respiration even though the oxygen level is little diminished.

Mechanics of Gill Ventilation

The mechanical sequence of respiration commences with water being drawn into the buccal cavity by opening the jaws and lowering the mouth floor. With the mouth then closed, water is forced through the gill slits and the mesh of laminae and secondary lamellae, by alternately raising the mouth floor (buccal pressure pump, increasing pressure before the gills) and then expanding the opercular cavity (opercular suction pump, reducing pressure behind the gills). Skin flaps inside the jaws prevent backflow of water out through the mouth, and a similar flap edging the gill cover permits only outflow from the opercular chamber (Fig.7). Coordination of these pumping movements maintains a high pressure in the buccal chamber and thus a continuous flow of water over the gills, although a "cough" can reverse water flow in response to pollutants.

Gill ventilation is monitored by proprioceptors and mechanoreceptors within the pseudobranch which initiate changes in both the volume of water pumped through the gills and the heart beat. These changes are in response to alterations in blood chemistry (oxygen , CO_2, and pH). The rate of pumping, and the volume of water passing through the gills increases with exercise and stress, such as depleted oxygen. An exercised rainbow trout might shift over three litres per minute for every kg of body weight (perhaps four times the resting flow). Smaller fish breathe more frequently than larger individuals. At rest, sticklebacks and minnows breathe up to 150 times per minute, much more frequently than sedentary species, such as bullheads and eels.

FIG.8: Mechanics of Gill Ventilation
[Adapted from: *Fish Health,* by Andrews, Excell and Carrington]

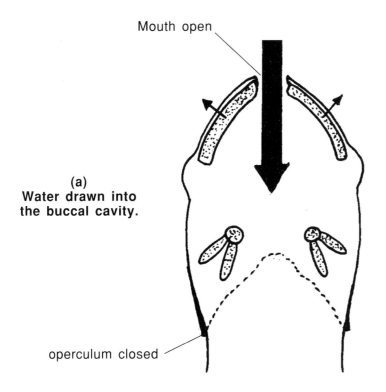

Mouth open

**(a)
Water drawn into
the buccal cavity.**

Opening of the jaws
and lowering of the floor
of the buccal cavity.

operculum closed

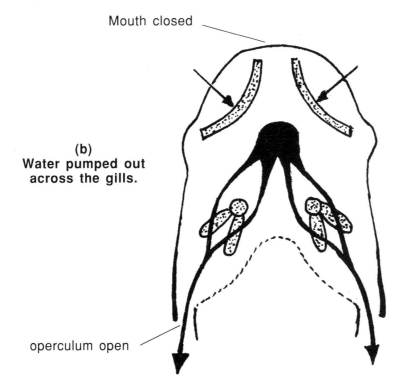

Mouth closed

**(b)
Water pumped out
across the gills.**

Closing of the jaws
and raising the floor
of the buccal cavity.

operculum open

Problems of "breathing" Water

Apart from enhancing the efficiency of absorption at the exchange interface, aquatic respiration must overcome the inherent problem of low dissolved oxygen content and the relatively hard work of pumping a much denser medium than air. At rest, a fish might need to use 10% of its oxygen uptake merely for the muscular activity of gill ventilation. Under circumstances of reduced oxygen availability, an attempt to compensate by increasing water flow might eventually be lethal.

Air Breathing

Under adverse conditions, fish may gulp at the surface, drawing the more highly oxygenated top layer of water and also air through the gills. A range of fresh and brackish water tropical teleosts can breathe air directly by accessory respiratory organs. Examples include a lung-like swimbladder in the freshwater "dogfish" *Umbra*, a gut modification in loach, and a vascularised gill cavity extension in the catfish *Clarias*. The anabantid fish (goramies, fighters) have a similarly vascularised labyrinth chamber above the gills, and may be seen in aquaria to take in air at the surface.

BUOYANCY

The body specific gravity of teleosts is somewhat heavier than that of the surrounding water (107% and 105% that of fresh and sea water respectively). However, fish can rise and stay in midwater by means of lift generated from two sources. The simpler method is called dynamic lift, achieved by inclining hydrofoils, especially the pectoral fins, when the body is in motion. A more economical method is that of static lift, which in the teleosts is normally achieved by means of the swimbladder.

Structure of the Swimbladder

The swimbladder has evolved from the primitive lung of lower bony fishes, and is a hydrostatic organ whereby neutral buoyancy is achieved and the fish can maintain itself in the water column without effort. It has developed as a dorsal diverticulum from the foregut, and possesses a typically thin wall. This wall has four layers - a lining epithelium, plain muscle, looser vascular connective tissue, and finally a tough fibrous outer layer, which also includes muscle and elastic tissue.

In the lower teleosts, the swimbladder retains an open pneumatic duct to the foregut, and is said to be physostomous. In the higher teleosts, there is no connection, and the swimbladder is described as physoclistous. In these physoclists, the swimbladder may be filled during larval development, when there is a temporary connection with the gut, or it may be inflated by gas secreted from cells within the sac. Most fish with a permanently physostomous swim bladder occur in fresh water. In such relatively shallow conditions, the swimbladder is easily refilled by swallowing without the need for gas secretion.

Functioning of the Swimbladder

The gas-filled swimbladder occupies about 7% of total body volume in freshwater fishes, and somewhat less (about 5%) in marine fishes. To maintain neutral buoyancy, it is necessary to alter the volume (inflation or deflation) as this changes with the water pressure at different depths (according to Boyle's Law). In lower teleosts, the gas content can be augmented by swimming to the surface and swallowing air which is then forced along the open pneumatic duct, or by voiding gases along the same route. Many cyprinids have a pneumatic bulb along the duct which can act as a pump for inflation. In the more specialised swimbladder, gas is secreted or absorbed through specialised regions of the wall (gas-gland and oval). These utilise a countercurrent system in a blood capillary bed (retia mirabilia), and their functioning depends on the area and blood flow.

The gas gland is in the anterior ventral part of the swimbladder. It occurs in many physostomes as well as physoclists. Liberation of gas from arterial blood in the capillaries of the gas gland into the lumen of the swimbladder results from an increase in blood acidity and operation of the Bohr and Root effects.

Gas is absorbed from the lumen of the swimbladder by exposure of the oval (so-called because of its usually oval outline), a capillary network supplied by the dorsal aorta and covered by thin epithelium. In many teleosts, exposure is controlled by circular or radial muscles, exposing or enclosing the absorptive surface on a rear part of the swimbladder. In others, such as sticklebacks and wrasses, the entire rear part of the swim bladder operates for this purpose and may be guarded by an impervious muscle diaphragm, while in the eel the resorptive capillary bed is associated with the pneumatic duct. In others, the oval is controlled by muscular action of the capillary walls or overlying epithelium. Absorbed gas is carried in venous blood via the cardinal veins to the heart, and excess may then be lost in solution at the gills. Nerve endings within the swimbladder wall respond to stretching and slackening, and both secretory and absorptive functions are controlled by the vagus.

Gas is held within the swimbladder by the impermeability of the walls. This is enhanced by a layer of guanine, a nitrogenous excretory product, which imparts a silvery appearance to the swimbladder. The gas components are oxygen, nitrogen and carbon dioxide. In shallow-water fishes, these gases are often in similar proportions to that of air, while in cyprinids only nitrogen is present. In physoclists, carbon dioxide predominates.

The swimbladder is often reduced in secondarily bottom-living teleosts, such as loach, catfish, gobies, flatfish and bullheads, in relation to their mode of life.

OSMOREGULATION AND EXCRETION

Tissue fluids in teleosts are intermediate in concentration between the extremes of fresh water and sea water, so that osmoregulatory problems are different in the two environments.

Marine Fishes

Marine teleosts are hyposmotic with respect to their environment (internal concentration about one quarter to one third that of the sea), with a resulting loss of water by osmosis through the gills. This is counteracted by continuous drinking of the sea water, at a rate of up to 0.5% body weight per hour. There is also some water loss in the urine, although this is only about one tenth of the volume produced by freshwater fish.

The intake of sea water results in salt absorption through the intestine, and even more sodium ions (approx. 5-10 times the amount drunk) diffuse into the blood through the gills. Since a fish cannot produce urine more concentrated than blood, its normal ionic balance can only be maintained by the active excretion of excess salt. This is achieved by special salt secreting "chloride" cells located mostly on the gill epithelium, which secrete sodium and chloride ions by active transport. These cells lie close together, and their action is believed to produce a localised area of high salt concentration, providing a local diffusion gradient that facilitates the passage of the excess salts into the sea. The kidney eliminates divalent ions, magnesium and sulphate, which account for about ten percent of the salts in sea water.

Freshwater Fishes

In fresh water the problem is reversed, the fish tissues being hyperosmotic to the surrounding water. There is thus a need to excrete vast amounts of water through the kidneys as copious dilute urine. The potential loss of solutes in the latter is reduced by the efficient resorption of sodium and chloride by the kidney tubules, as well as reduced permeability of the gills. Any net loss of ions is made up by active transport from the fresh water across the gills. Each ion is exchanged independently, Na^+ for NH_4^+ and H^+, Cl^- for HCO_3^- (NH_4^+ and HCO_3^- being excretory products).The same cell type (an acidophil) is responsible for this process in both marine and freshwater fish.

Euryhaline Fishes

There are also fishes which are euryhaline (i.e. tolerant of a wide range of salinities) or which migrate from the sea to fresh water, or vice versa, during their life history. Species like eels, sticklebacks and some killifish take 1-2 days to adapt their excretory pattern to suit their new environment. The Killifish, *Fundulus*, can live in freshwater as well as in hypersaline pools of up to 128 ppt (seawater is about 35 ppt). At salinities in excess of 60 ppt, a water loss of about 5% is tolerated, with a resulting increase in blood concentration. Endocrine changes during this transition include thyroid activity in salmon descending to the sea.

Nitrogenous Excretion

The kidneys in teleosts are elongate structures, closely applied to the roof of the abdominal cavity. Basically paired, they vary in the degree and pattern of fusion, which is almost complete in salmonids, but incomplete along the mid-line in many cyprinids. The anterior part, or head of the kidney, is haemopoietic, while the more posterior part is excretory The structure of the nephron differs between marine, brackish and freshwater species, reflecting their different physiological requirements.

It is important to realise that the gills, and not the kidneys, are the most important site of nitrogenous excretion in fishes. The main excretory product in fish is ammonia (fish are thus said to be *ammonotelic*), the final nitrogenous product of amino-acid metabolism. It is highly soluble, and is rapidly lost through the gills. In carp, the gills lose 6-10 times more nitrogen than the kidneys, and 90% of this is in the form of ammonia, the rest mostly urea.

NERVOUS SYSTEM

A detailed discussion of the nervous system in fish is beyond the scope of this manual. Basically the fish brain comprises three major parts, the forebrain, midbrain, and hindbrain, which differ in relative proportions according to mode of life of the species. Relative brain size in fish may vary from about 0.1% body weight in some predators, to up to about 1% in the African freshwater mormyrids. The brain normally does not fill the braincase cavity of the skull and is surrounded by a simple meningeal membrane.

There are 10 cranial nerves and the spinal cord gives off segmentally arranged nerve roots as in higher vertebrates. There is a well developed autonomic nervous system.

Sense Organs

The senses of teleosts are vision, smell, taste, hearing and "distance-touch". There are the obvious special sense organs, the eye, the ear (not visible externally), the lateral-line system, the olfactory sac with nostrils, as well as taste and smell buds over the skin. Free nerve endings also occur in the skin and the swimbladder, and these are sensitive to touch, temperature, and pressure.

Energy stimuli for the teleost may be electromagnetic (light and electrical) and mechanical (sound and vibrations). In water, higher frequency compression waves from mechanical disturbances are monitored by the inner ear as "hearing", and those of lower frequency by the lateral-line system as "vibrations", a "distance-touch sense" for short-range use.

Smell/Taste

In water, the distinction between smell (long range detection of objects, from molecules diffused or carried by currents) and taste (stimulation by molecules on contact with the object) is less obvious than in air. There are generally paired olfactory sacs on the snout, water passing over the receptors during swimming or by pumping action. These are very sensitive to amino-acids, and some species have been shown to have well developed powers of discrimination between conspecifics and other organisms such as water plants. Homing salmon may distinguish their own rivers by smell. Within species, chemicals generated for communication (pheromones) include special sex steroids for courtship (such as from the mesorchial gland of gobioid fish) and alarm substances from the damaged skin of minnows and many other cyprinids.

Taste-buds, similar to those of the olfactory lining, occur on the lips, mouth, pharynx and gill arches. They are also distributed over the head and fins, and in many species occur all over the body, but particularly on special structures like barbels, which can be highly mobile as in red mullet.

Hearing

The fish ear lies within the skull and consists of 3 interconnecting sacs. These are the utriculus (together with the semicircular canals responsible for balance) and the sacculus and lagena (sensitive to vibrations).

Teleosts overall can distinguish tones between 16 and 7000 cps. This is enhanced in many modern teleosts by using the swimbladder as a resonating chamber. Various kinds of ear-swimbladder connection are found. By far the most important group of freshwater teleosts (Ostariophysi : characins [tetras, piranhas], carps, catfish, etc.) have a system in which the swimbladder is hour-glass shaped, and the anterior chamber is linked to the inner ear by a chain of three small bones (Weberian ossicles) derived from parts of the anterior vertebrae, which transmit vibrations to the fluid (perilymph) around the inner ear. Fish without a swimbladder have a hearing limit of about 400 Hz; with a swimbladder unconnected to the ear it is 520 Hz, but with swimbladder and Weberian ossicles the limit is increased to 5000-7000 Hz (to 10000 cps). They also have sharper hearing and better pitch discrimination. Fish in general are deaf to high frequency sounds (>20,000 cps).

It is thought that communication by sound between conspecifics may be important in stimulating behaviour patterns associated with shoaling, feeding, and reproduction.

Vibration

Low frequency compression waves are monitored by the lateral line system, a series of perforated tubes under the skin over head and body, notably along the lateral midline of the body. It enables the recognition of disturbances in currents caused by conspecifics or other species (prey or predators), as well as those rebounding from static obstacles.

Electroreception

Electrical stimuli are conducted in water, and a number of teleosts have electric organs derived from modified muscle tissue. Weakly electric fish, such as African mormyrids and South American knifefish (gymnotids), generate fields for electrolocation of obstacles and prey in turbid water, as well as for communication. More powerful electric fish (such as the Electric "Eel", *Electrophorus*), generate high potentials (up to 500 Volts in the latter) for stunning prey or attackers.

Vision

The teleosts show a much greater variety of eye modifications than land vertebrates, because light environments are more diverse in water. Light wavelength, colours and even the pattern of combination of letters can be discriminated among teleosts.

The basic structure of the eye-ball and humoral contents is similar throughout the vertebrates. The similarity in refractive index of water (1.33) to that of the cornea means that the lens in fishes is responsible for focussing the image on the retina. The ideal lens shape is spherical, such that the lens tends to protrude through the pupil, producing a short focal length and the highest effective refractive index (1.65) in vertebrates. Both the cornea or lens may be tinted. Accommodation (exact definition by adjusting focus) is achieved by moving the lens rather than changing its shape.

There are also at least 40 species of cave fishes (about a third catfish), with eye reduction to the extent of blindness.

BEHAVIOUR

Behaviour patterns result from interaction between external stimuli, genetic and phenotypic constraints, and the internal state of the fish. Part of fish behaviour is predominantly instinctive, in which a fixed response (e.g. an escape action), to a particular set of stimuli (e.g. the detection of a predator), is genetically determined. Instinctive behaviour may be modified by learning on the part of an individual fish.

The internal state of the fish can affect behaviour by inducing a "consummatory drive". Thus, a physiological state without food in the stomach, and low levels of blood constituents, will result in "hunger" and a feeding drive. In the sexually mature fish, blood levels of sex hormones are associated with reproductive behaviour. Behaviour patterns may therefore exhibit marked seasonality, as well as daily rhythms in connection with light or tidal cycles.

A variety of physical stimuli are known to elicit behavioural responses, such as geotaxis and orientation. Rheotaxis (behaviour with respect to current flow), and associated optomotor responses, are manifest in station-keeping fishes of running water. Reaction to directional light is easily observed in aquaria, and an aberrant inversion of the body to light and gravity is shown by the habitually upside-down Catfish, *Synodontis* sp. Feeding or homing behaviour can result from olfaction of minute traces of organic substances.

The biological environment elicits behaviour with respect to conspecifics and to other species in the ecosystem. The latter may be the subject of feeding behaviour, avoidance, or agonistic defence of territory. Feeding typically involves the locomotor patterns of searching, detection, capture and ingestion. In some instances, there are commensal behaviour patterns with other species (e.g. Anemone fish *Amphiprion* with a sea-anemone, the watchman goby *Cryptocentrus* in the burrow of a prawn).

Behavioural interaction with conspecifics is often territorial and, of course, includes reproduction. It is most evident in shoal formation, seen in many midwater fish species. Shoals, although closely integrated, are leaderless, and are believed to serve a protective function against predators as well as, for some species, a part of spawning procedure.

Between conspecifics, it is possible to identify fixed patterns of display (characterised by body and fin posture and movement). These "sign stimuli" are themselves initiated by those from the other fish. Sensory response may be visual, depending on the sight of special configurations of posture and movement (e.g. fin spreading and body arching). The display by the male Siamese Fighter to its reflection in a mirror can be easily arranged to observe this. In many teleosts, visual stimuli may be reinforced by sound production and pheromones. Interactive behaviour often leads to the establishment of dominance or pecking order in a group of captive fish, typically in order of size, and this may have noticeable effects on appearance (submissive behaviour and paler coloration), feeding, growth performance, and reproductive success.

Reproductive behaviour, and its associated territoriality, is the most widely studied of the behaviour patterns in ornamental fishes, especially the cichlids, anabantids, and sticklebacks. Reproductive behaviour varies in complexity, from promiscuous spawning in goldfish to a whole sequence of territoriality, courtship and brood care in cichlids. Nest preparation among ornamental fishes may involve cleaning of a stone or leaf surface, excavation (as in cichlids), or blowing a bubble nest (as in anabantid species). Behaviour sequences of courtship are often based on special nuptial coloration of the mature fish (e.g: red breast of sticklebacks, and the marked dimorphism of guppies). Some behaviour patterns have become ritualised, being similar to those which serve a useful function in another situation, and seemingly irrelevant in the reproductive context (e.g. stickleback digging in a territorial dispute). Species-specificity of behaviour and sexual sign stimuli contribute to reproductive isolation between species. After spawning, brood care, best seen among cichlids, may involve fanning of eggs and defence against predators, which in some cases continues for a short time after hatching. Some cichlids are mouthbrooders and in others, such as discus, the young feed on parental skin mucus.

Instinctive behaviour patterns can be modified by learning, as when male guppies learn to restrict their attempts at mating to the female sex. The ability of fish to learn is soon evident to aquarium keepers, when fish congregate for feeding on approach or disturbance to the tank. The catfish, *Ameirus*, can associate food with a whistle, or even words. Conditioned reflexes in fish have been used to investigate powers of sensory discrimination, such as colour vision in the presentation of unpalatable food. On average, about 30 presentations are needed, and the reflex may survive intervals of up to several weeks. More elaborate learning is demonstrated by sticklebacks and cichlids, which come to avoid glass interposed between them and food, and in maze learning by sunfish. If the theory is correct, salmon learn the odours of their birth streams, and remember them when homing after some years at sea.

ENDOCRINOLOGY

The basic plan of the teleost endocrine system is similar to that of higher vertebrates. Peculiarities include the diffuse thyroid and the primitive separation of the adrenal components, as well as glands that are restricted to fish, whose function is little understood.

Pituitary:

Similar to that in higher vertebrates. The hormones produced stimulate other endocrine organs (e.g. thyroid, gonads, etc.), and influence physiological processes (e.g. melanophore behaviour and osmoregulation). Pituitary extracts may be used to stimulate spawning in cultivated species.

Thyroid:

Thyroid follicles are dispersed through connective tissue around the ventral aorta, and sometimes even as far afield as the eye, hepatic veins and kidney. The hormone is an iodinated dipeptide (thyroxine), which stimulates metabolism.

Interrenal:

There is no combined adrenal gland in the vast majority of fish, and this equivalent of the mammalian adrenal cortex is found as strands of interrenal tissue in the anterior kidney, associated with major blood vessels. Corticosteroid hormones are produced, acting similarly to those of higher vertebrates.

The mineralocorticoids (eg. aldosterone) may be important in controlling ionic balance, especially sodium transfer across the gills.

Suprarenal:

The adrenal medulla of higher vertebrates is represented by suprarenal or chromaffin tissue, often in clumps related to the anterior kidney, sympathetic ganglia, and sometimes actually in contact with interrenal tissue. It produces sympathomimetic hormones such as adrenaline and noradrenaline, involved in the initial stress response.

Endocrine Pancreas:

Islets of Langerhans are distributed throughout the pancreas, itself a somewhat variable organ in fishes, and may be grouped into a large islet, the Brockman body. Within the capsule of each islet, both glucagon and insulin producing cells occur, although the action of these fish hormones may differ from the mammalian properties.

Ultimobranchial glands:

These are tracts of cells situated below the gullet, between the sinus venosus and abdominal cavity, formed from the fifth gill arch of the embryo. Corresponding to the mammalian parathyroid, the ultimobranchial glands control serum calcium levels.

Corpuscles of Stannius:

These are paired secretory bodies on the surface of the kidney, involved in calcium metabolism and possibly osmoregulation.

Urophysis:

This is a small swelling of the spinal cord at its rear tip, well vascularised and draining into the renal portal system. It consists of neurosecretory axons from the cord, reminiscent of those in the hypothalamus of the brain/pituitary link.

Gonads:

Steroids are produced from interstitial tissue of the testis, and follicular tissue of the ovary. Nuptial coloration and other secondary sexual characters result from male steroid activity. In male gobies, the interstitial tissue may be aggregated into a prominent mesorchial gland along the sperm duct side of the testis, the secretions of which serve as pheromones. In female teleosts, oestrogens are essential for the production of yolk proteins by the liver, to be subsequently incorporated into the maturing ovary.

Pseudobranch and Choroid Body:

The pseudobranch is a reddish vascularised body on the inner face of the opercle, and is derived from the hyoidean gill arch. In conjunction with this there is a similarly vascularised choroid body in the eye. The functions of the pseudobranch may be endocrine as well as hyperoxygenation of blood for the retina, since its blood supply is efferent from the first functional gill arch.

STRESS

This is an environmental stimulus which extends the adaptive response of the fish beyond its range of "normal" functioning, to the extent that metabolic performance and the chances of survival are reduced under chronic conditions.

The response by the fish to stress has been termed the **General Adaption Syndrome (G.A.S.)**. It is a sequence of physiological changes which ensue regardless of the nature of the initial stimulus. Stress can be anything outside the fish's norm of experience - temperature changes, pollutants, handling, social effects, or disease, and is an important factor in fish culture, where the overall environment may be highly artificial.

It is convenient to distinguish three stages in G.A.S.:

1. Primary : Neural and neuroendocrine responses, involving the pituitary (ACTH), interrenal (corticosteroids), and chromaffin (catecholamines) tissues. This is essentially alarm.

2. Secondary : The physiological consequences of (i), with changes in blood chemistry, metabolic rate, and osmoregulation. This has been termed the "phase of resistance".

3. Tertiary : The effects are widespread and include behavioural changes, decreased growth rate, increased susceptibility to disease, and impairment of gonad maturation. This leads to progressive exhaustion, debility and death.

REPRODUCTION

Gonads and Gametogenesis

The reproductive organs (gonads) of fish are typically paired, elongate structures suspended by a ligament from the roof of the abdominal cavity, flanking or lying below the swimbladder when this is present. In the poeciliids, they are fused into one structure.

The gametes are formed by the usual gametogenetic divisions to halve chromosome number, although, in the egg, the last occurs usually only after sperm entry. Gonad maturation involves a substantial increase in bulk, especially for the ovaries, which may reach 70% of body weight. The testes are usually much smaller, but achieve almost 12% of body weight in some species.

Oocyte development begins as a primary phase, independent of pituitary hormone control. Once the oocytes reach a certain critical size, they commence vitellogenesis (yolk deposition) and the maturing oocytes greatly enlarge, this process requiring the pituitary secretion of gonadotrophin. Further ripening occurs and eventually there is final maturation, usually involving water uptake, considerably increasing the volume. This may involve the entire developing oocyte population synchronously, or successive groups, in the case of a repeat-spawning species, during a breeding season. The number of eggs produced (fecundity) is normally a positive exponential function of body size. In fisheries, it is often useful to categorise the reproductive state of the fish from the gross appearance of the gonads. The terms commonly used are "immature virgin", "ripening", "running ripe", "spent", and "recovering spent".

Sexual Dimorphism

Basic external differences between the sexes may involve contrasting shape of a urogenital papilla, and, in viviparous species, various copulatory organs possessed by the male. There are many examples of sexual dimorphism involving intensity of coloration and fin development (eg Siamese fighting fish), body proportions and absolute size, and even special organs such as white nuptial tubercles (carps).

Behaviour

The essential act of fertilisation normally requires a behavioural sequence of mating. Actual spawning may occur in a shoal or with elaborate behaviour, involving a sequence of courtship and display, often centring on a territory and a nest. After fertilisation, the eggs of many species (such as carp, characins and killifish) are then abandoned by the parents. Those species producing fewer demersal eggs may perform some degree of egg care, while others even care for their brood following hatching (e.g: cichlids). Male pipefish and seahorses "gestate" the eggs after fertilisation, while mouthbrooding and viviparity may be viewed as other extreme strategies.

Sexuality

The majority of teleosts are gonochoristic (with two sexes) but in some families, such as the wrasses, hermaphroditism is frequent, usually with females changing into males (protogyny) via a transient ovotestis. In a number of teleosts, sex is associated with heterokary (females XX, males XY), but this may be reversed or not evident, and sex change may be effected by hormone treatment. Parthenogenesis (development from an unfertilised egg) and gynogenesis (sperm penetration of oocyte, but not nuclear fusion before development) can occur. The latter process is found in some poeciliids, which are all female species, and which require the entry of sperm from males of related species into the egg cytoplasm to stimulate further development. Development of the egg can also be induced by artificial means without fusion between female and male nuclei.

Embryonic Development

Embryonic development is most obviously influenced by temperature. Within the range of tolerance of the species, the rate of development quickens with increasing temperature. Temperature also affects the fixation of serial (meristic) features, such as the number of vertebrae and fin-rays, in early development. Other environmental factors affect development. Eggs of various salmonids produce larger embryos and hatch earlier at higher oxygen content and faster water flow.

The degree of growth and differentiation achieved at hatching varies greatly between species, and many teleosts have a distinctive larval stage before adopting a juvenile version of the definitive adult form. Planktonic larvae float by means of oil globules, high water content, or elongate processes such as fins or spines. Between hatching and this metamorphosis, the larva is described as a prolarva, while still possessing a yolk sac, and as a postlarva, between complete absorption of the yolk sac and metamorphosis. Many species then hatch as postlarvae. Others change from a yolk carrying prolarva into the juvenile form without a distinct metamorphosis, and, as in salmonids, these are termed alevins. The rate of growth in young teleosts is influenced most conspicuously by temperature, food supply, and reproduction, but a host of environmental factors may have a complex effect. These may include salinity, photoperiod, living space, and biological influences, such as social interaction with conspecifics.

Acknowledgement:– Many thanks to John Wiley and Sons, inc. for permission to adapt the original diagrams of Figures 2, 4 and 5 in this chapter.

CHAPTER TWO # WATER QUALITY

Lydia A. Brown

Water is the universal solvent. It is also the only habitat in which fish can survive, and it is essential to all plant and animal life in a variety of ways. Under natural conditions water does not exist in a pure state, and so the additional chemicals and organic compounds present in solution will be discussed with respect to their ability to sustain fish life. Fish live in a variety of habitats, and so only general comments can be made regarding the physical and chemical factors relating to water quality.

PHYSICAL PROPERTIES

Density

At 4°C, the density of water is 1.00, while at warmer temperatures it becomes less dense, or lighter. Ice, too, is less dense than water, and if it were not for this fact, water would freeze from the bottom up, thus preventing aquatic life from existing in temperate or arctic areas. Temperature, pressure and the presence of dissolved substances all change the density of water.

Water currents

These are classified as horizontal, vertical, returning or density currents. They are extremely important in aeration of the water and the distribution of plant nutrients, etc.

Temperature and Stratification

Water has the highest specific heat (amount of heat required to raise the temperature of 1g of a substance by 1°C) of any known substance. It therefore changes temperature more slowly than the surrounding air or soil. Changes in water temperature can also affect water density.

Water stratifies in large open masses very easily. In static water (e.g. a pond), differences in temperature cause a layering effect. This is most pronounced in Summer and Winter. The layers are called:

1. The epilimnion - the top layer
2. The thermocline - the transitional layer
3. The hypolimnion - the bottom layer

Shallow waters may only show the thermocline characteristics; cool water tends to remain on the bottom in hot weather, whereas the warmest waters will be on the bottom in freezing weather. Considerable force is required to displace the bottom layer if the temperature difference between the layers is great. Prolonged stratification, particularly in organically rich waters, renders the bottom unsuitable for life which requires oxygen. Certain weather conditions (e.g. winds, heavy rain, etc.), tend to break up the stratification. This is also achieved by the use of pumps and filters in small ponds.

28

Light penetration

This is very important for photosynthesis, and affects temperature and oxygen relationships in water. It is itself influenced by the turbidity of the water, the intensity and duration of sunlight, the amount of wind action, and algal/plant growth etc.

Turbidity is caused by suspended materials of various kinds, and greatly affects light penetration. It has an important influence on heat exchange which also affects the type and amount of plant life in the pond.

CHEMICAL PROPERTIES

Alkalinity

Total alkalinity is the total concentration of bases, carbonates (CO_3^{2-}) and bicarbonates (HCO_3^-) in water, expressed as parts per million (ppm), or milligrams per litre (mg/1), of equivalent calcium carbonate ($CaCO_3$).

Another way to think of alkalinity is in terms of resistance to pH change. The amount of acid required to cause a specific change in pH in a given volume, increases as the total alkalinity increases (i.e. it is a measure of the buffering capacity of water).

The principle anions of almost all freshwaters are bicarbonates, carbonates, hydroxides, phosphates, sulphates and chlorides .In most natural waters bicarbonates and sometimes carbonates are present. These salts are hydrolysed in solution because of the weakness of carbonic acid (H_2CO_3), with the production of hydroxyl ions and consequent rises in pH.

$$HCO_3^- + H_2O \rightleftharpoons H_2CO_3 + OH^-$$

The most useful method of measuring the concentrations of combined anions of weak acids is the acid combining capacity or alkalinity. The sample is titrated with standard acid until the above equilibrium has moved completely to the right.

Total alkalinity is determined by titrating a sample of water with standardised acid to the colour change of methyl orange. The best fish production is generally associated with a total alkalinity of 100 to 120 ppm. Alkalinity will vary on a daily, and a seasonal basis. Because of the influence of carbon dioxide, the pH of pond waters is lowest at or near dawn and highest in the afternoon. This diurnal fluctuation is greatest when phytoplankton growth is rapid. Waters with moderate, or high, bicarbonate concentrations have greater carbon dioxide reserves, and so such fluctuations in pH are often less than in waters with low bicarbonate concentrations.

The addition of calcium carbonate (limestone) to acid waters will serve to increase the pH as it dissolves and introduces carbonate ions to the water. As the carbonate concentration increases the solubility of calcium carbonate may be exceeded resulting in precipitation and a moderation of the rise in pH.

Alkalinity is a most important parameter in marine aquaria where the water is prepared from a commercial, artificial sea salt mix. Many of the commercially available salt mixes rely on the presence of alkalinity in the domestic water supply to provide the buffering capacity required to maintain the pH at about 8.2. In soft water areas this is not sufficient, and catastrophic falls in pH can result. It is as important to measure the alkalinity of marine aquaria as the pH.

Total Harness

This refers to the concentration of divalent metal ions (e.g: calcium, magnesium, iron and aluminium) in water expressed as equivalent milligrams per litre of calcium carbonate. The part of the total hardness which is equivalent to the alkalinity is termed the **carbonate hardness** or **temporary hardness**.

Hardness should generally be greater than 10 mg/litre as $CaCO_3$.

pH of Water

The pH is an expression of the relationship between H^+ and OH^- ions present in water. A value of 7 is neutral, while values less than 7 are acid, and greater than 7 are alkaline. Each one unit change in pH value represents a 10 fold change in hydrogen ion concentration. Fish prefer a pH of 7.0 to 7.5, but various species may occupy habitat niches over the range of 6.5 to 8.5. At a pH of less than 6, fish may still survive, but growth will be impeded. Some fish may still *survive* at a pH of 5.

Hydroxides are involved in water alkalinity and result when plants extract bound CO_2 from carbonates of calcium, sodium, and magnesium (probably more of the latter two). It is an active toxicant in lime sterilisation, and begins to affect fish life directly at a pH of 10-11.

Buffer effects in water

Buffer effects are the result of ionisation and reaction of buffer salts which are formed by weak acids. Thus calcium carbonate will buffer chemical changes associated with carbonic acid. Water supplies which have a lot of buffering capacity are generally easier to manage since drastic changes in water quality are buffered by these substances. Not all effects are desirable, as they may decrease the effect of disease and herbicide treatments, etc.

GAS RELATIONSHIPS OF WATER

General Properties

Equilibria become established under a given set of conditions with some of the gas entering water and an equal amount leaving. More gas can be dissolved at low temperatures compared with high temperatures. An increase in dissolved solids decreases the solubility of gases. The amount of water vapour a gas contains affects its solubility in water. Surface agitation or wave action increases the rate of change.

Oxygen

The main sources of oxygen are from plant photosynthesis and diffusion from the atmosphere. The latter is very limited and only occurs at the water surface, although it can be improved by using mechanical aerators, air stones, and fountain sprays. For static water, photosynthesis is the principle source of oxygen. Oxygen concentrations vary diurnally, such that low levels occur at night, when previously photosynthesising organisms are respiring and consume oxygen.

If too much oxygen is present, gas bubble disease can occur, especially in young fish. This can occur with the over zealous use of aerators in warm weather, when the solubility of oxygen is reduced.

The amount of CO_2 and ammonia present influences the concentration of oxygen in the water below which fish may die. Bacterial action probably represents the greatest influence in oxygen removal under pond conditions. As a general rule of thumb, a dissolved oxygen concentration (D.O.) which falls below 6 ppm and/or 70% saturation for cool and cold water species is dangerous. Most species of warm water fishes are not stressed until the dissolved oxygen falls below 4 ppm.

Carbon Dioxide

Carbon dioxide (CO_2) may be harmful if there is more than 10ppm in the water. Reserve amounts of carbon dioxide are present in bicarbonates, carbonates and in inorganic forms. It is essential for plant growth and is a limiting factor to their growth in soft acid water.

Sources of carbon dioxide include diffusion from the atmosphere, inflowing ground water, decomposition of organic matter, and respiration of living organisms. Decomposition of organic matter is probably the most important source in most ponds. Losses of CO_2 are caused by photosynthesis, precipitation of carbonates, diffusion into the atmosphere, and chemical combination.

NITROGENOUS COMPOUNDS

Ammonia

Ammonia is seldom present in appreciable amounts if conditions are favourable for green plant growth. A level of 1 ppm total ammonia nitrogen is an indication of pollution and 2-3 ppm is cause for concern.

The toxicity of ammonia is greater when the pH and temperature are high and the D.O. is low. High levels can be reduced by flushing, dilution, uptake by plants, and by aeration.

Sources of ammonia are metabolic waste, feed residues, decaying plants, inflowing water and nitrogen fixing plants. The natural path of the conversion of ammonia to nitrogen is given below

FIG.1: The Nitrogen Cycle

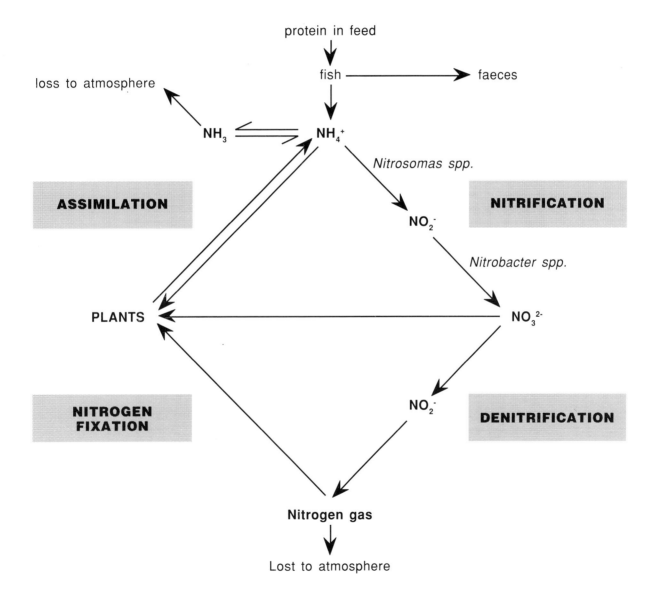

Proteins in the food are an important source of nitrogen in fish production. Bacteria decompose organic matter and ammonia into nitrite, and then further to nitrate, which is readily assimilated into new tissues by plants. Some nitrates are lost to sediments.

The Total ammonia nitrogen is the sum of that present as both the ionized ammonium ion(NH_4^+), as well as unionized ammonia (NH_3). The unionized ammonia is toxic to fish, whereas ionized ammonium ion is non toxic. In solution, ammonia forms the following equilibrium:

Increasing pH and/or Temperature.

$$NH_3 + H_2O \rightleftharpoons NH_4^+ + OH^-$$

Decreasing pH and/or Temperature.

The pH and water temperature affect the equilibrium of the equation as indicated. Reference to Table 1 will facilitate the calculation of the % unionised ammonia from the Total Ammonia Nitrogen (the parameter generally measured in water).

The maximum safe concentration of unionised ammonia is 0.025 mg/1. Levels of unionised ammonia, which may not necessarily be fatal, will result in chronic stress, with the subsequent development of gill and kidney tissue damage.

High levels of ammonia are generally a sign of overfeeding and/or overstocking, and can be alleviated by reducing these factors, or by increasing water flow.

Table 1:
The Percentage of unionised ammonia in aqueous
solutions at different pH values and temperatures.

pH	Temperature (°C)														
	4	6	8	10	12	14	16	18	20	22	24	26	28	30	32
7.0	0.11	0.13	0.16	0.18	0.22	0.25	0.29	0.34	0.39	0.46	0.52	0.60	0.69	0.80	0.91
7.2	0.18	0.21	0.25	0.29	0.34	0.40	0.46	0.54	0.62	0.72	0.83	0.96	1.10	1.26	1.44
7.4	0.29	0.34	0.40	0.46	0.54	0.63	0.73	0.85	0.98	1.14	1.31	1.50	1.73	1.98	2.26
7.6	0.45	0.53	0.63	0.73	0.86	1.00	1.16	1.34	1.55	1.79	2.06	2.36	2.71	3.10	3.53
7.8	0.72	0.84	0.99	1.16	1.35	1.57	1.82	2.11	2.44	2.81	3.22	3.70	4.23	4.82	5.48
8.0	1.13	1.33	1.56	1.82	2.12	2.47	2.86	3.30	3.81	4.38	5.02	5.74	6.54	7.43	8.42
8.2	1.79	2.10	2.45	2.86	3.32	3.85	4.45	5.14	5.90	6.76	7.72	8.80	9.98	11.29	12.72
8.4	2.80	3.28	3.83	4.45	5.17	5.97	6.88	7.90	9.04	10.31	11.71	13.26	14.95	16.78	18.77
8.6	4.37	5.10	5.93	6.88	7.95	9.14	10.48	11.97	13.61	15.41	17.37	19.50	21.78	24.22	26.80
8.8	6.75	7.85	9.09	10.48	12.04	13.76	15.66	17.73	19.98	22.41	25.00	27.74	30.62	33.62	36.72
9.0	10.30	11.90	13.68	15.67	17.82	20.18	22.73	25.46	28.36	31.40	34.56	37.83	41.16	44.53	47.91
9.2	15.39	17.63	20.08	22.73	25.58	28.61	31.80	35.12	38.55	42.04	45.57	49.09	52.58	55.99	59.31
9.4	22.38	25.33	28.67	31.80	35.26	38.84	42.49	46.18	49.85	53.48	57.02	60.45	63.73	66.85	69.79
9.6	31.36	34.96	38.68	42.49	46.33	50.16	53.94	57.62	61.17	64.56	67.77	70.78	73.58	76.17	78.55
9.8	42.00	46.00	50.00	53.94	57.78	61.47	64.99	68.31	71.40	74.28	76.92	79.33	81.53	83.51	85.30
10.0	53.44	57.45	61.31	64.98	68.44	71.66	74.63	77.35	79.83	82.07	84.08	85.88	87.49	88.92	90.19
10.2	64.53	68.15	71.52	74.63	77.46	80.03	82.34	84.41	86.25	87.88	89.33	90.60	91.73	92.71	93.38

Ref: Emerson K., Russo R. C., Lund R. E. and Thurston R. V. 1975
Aqueous ammonia equilibrium calculations effect of pH and temperature.
J Fish. Res. Bd. Can. **32:** 2379 – 2383

Nitrites

High nitrite concentrations (greater than 1.0 mg/1) can kill fish within 24 hours if the chloride concentration present is inadequate to afford protection.

Methaemoglobinaemia is caused by high nitrite values in fresh water. The fish die, basically from asphyxiation, since oxygen cannot bind onto methaemoglobin. The toxicity of nitrites can be countered by adding sodium chloride, since chloride is taken up by the gills in preference to nitrite. A minimum ratio of chlorides to nitrites that will afford protection is 5:1.

Nitrites appear to be less toxic in hard water than in soft water.

Nitrates

Nitrates are the least toxic of all the nitrogenous compounds, 1000 to 2000 mg/1 nitrate nitrogen being generally toxic to fish.

MISCELLANEOUS SOLUTES

Calcium

Calcium is found in combination with carbonates, bicarbonates, sulphates, chlorides, nitrates or hydroxides. It is the major element in water hardness, and calcium salts generally have a low solubility.

It is also an important component of the buffer system ,a micronutrient for plants, and a mineral required by animals. High levels reduce the availability of phosphates and iron, and also affect the action of several herbicides.

Chlorides

The amounts generally found even up to 1000 to 2000 ppm are not an influencing factor in fish health. Chlorides and sulphates are major salts in ground waters where a noticeable brine content is present.

Hydrogen Sulphide

Hydrogen sulphide is a poisonous gas and is highly soluble in water. It is produced when organic matter decays anaerobically. Concentrations of more than 0.3 ppm are cause for concern.

Hydroxides

Hydroxides are involved in water alkalinity and result when plants extract bound CO_2 from carbonates of calcium, sodium and magnesium. It is an active toxicant in lime sterilisation and begins to affect fish life directly at a pH of 10-11.

Iron

Iron is common in ground water as the soluble ferrous (Fe^{2+}) salt. It oxidises to the ferric (Fe^{3+}) form when it is aerated. The ferric form is relatively insoluble and precipitates. The iron influences the availability of phosphates, and mechanically clogs gills of fishes held in water carrying noticeable amounts of the ferric form. More than 0.3 ppm can be a cause for concern.

Magnesium

Magnesium has a similar role to calcium and is frequently associated with it in rock formations, although the salts of magnesium are more soluble than those of calcium. It contributes to the total hardness of water; however it is less desirable than calcium, being a factor in highly alkaline pH development (although to a lesser extent than sodium). It is an essential micronutrient for growth of green aquatic plants.

Manganese

Manganese is generally associated with iron, and has a chemical oxygen demand as monovalent $Mn+$. It has proven to be toxic to trout under some conditions.

Nitrogen

As a gas, nitrogen is inert and non toxic. It has caused gas bubble disease when present in large amounts in ground water supplies. It is unavailable to plants, except by a special group of nitrogen fixing plants.

Phosphate

Phosphate is normally present in minute amounts (less than 0.1 ppm). It is a macronutrient for green plant growth. It tends to be removed by bottom mud, and is usually the first plant nutrient to become limiting in plant growth.

Potassium

Potassium is non toxic at levels normally found in water. It is a macronutrient for green plant growth. It is present to some extent in many soils and ground water. Potassium is not limiting to plant growth as often as phosphorous or nitrogen.

Sodium

Sodium is highly soluble and is not really toxic to fishes. It is important in buffer systems when associated with bicarbonates and carbonates. High alkalinities are related to an abundance of sodium carbonate and bicarbonate in fertile water situations.

Sulphates

Sulphates are common in water supplies of many parts of the country and are often combined with calcium, magnesium, iron and aluminium. They are seldom a direct factor in the well being of fish. A point to note is that more than 100 ppm may affect the durability of concrete structures used to hold fish.

Zinc

Zinc salts are usually very soluble. It has been reported as toxic to fish at a level of 0.04 ppm in soft water. Fish eggs and sac fry are sensitive to low levels. Calcium minimises the toxic effects, whilst copper synergises them. New galvanised pipe or containers carrying soft, acid water may pick up enough zinc to be toxic to fishes.

Acknowledgements

Much of this chapter was taken from notes prepared by Dr T Wellborn and his colleagues at the Mississippi Agriculture, Forestry Extension Service (MAFES) to whom acknowledgement is made.

Thanks are also due to Mr K Digby of New Technology Ltd.

CHAPTER THREE

AQUARIUM FISHKEEPING

Chris Andrews

TYPES OF AQUARIUM FISHKEEPING

Aquarium fishkeeping can be broadly divided into freshwater and marine, coldwater (unheated) and tropical (heated).

In unheated, freshwater aquaria, fish such as goldfish, carp and other coldwater species are kept, whilst a huge range of tropical freshwater fish are available for the heated freshwater aquarium. Living plants are a common decorative feature in tropical freshwater tanks, although less so in coldwater aquaria. Artificial (plastic) plants are also available.

A range of coral reef fish, invertebrates and even certain seaweeds (macro-algae) are kept in heated marine aquaria, and there is some interest in the maintenance of local (i.e. temperate) inshore fish and invertebrates in unheated or even chilled marine aquaria.

On occasion certain species of tropical estuarine fish are kept in heated brackish water aquaria containing (perhaps) one quarter to one third strength seawater.

So long as certain guidelines are followed, the establishment and successful maintenance of coldwater or topical freshwater aquaria is relatively straightforward. Marine aquaria are rather more troublesome for the novice fishkeeper and usually recommended for relatively experienced aquarists.

IMPORTANT CONSIDERATIONS

Siting an aquarium

Choosing a suitable site for an aquarium is very important. The aquarium must be away from room heaters, draughts and direct sunlight, which may all encourage fluctuations in water temperature and often (in the case of sunlight) precipitate unsightly algal growth.

A convenient power source is likely to be needed for most aquaria and one 13-amp socket should be sufficient for a single tank. Water will have to be brought to, and taken from the tank, usually in buckets. Aquaria can be very heavy, each gallon of water weighing 10lbs. Therefore, the aquarium will have to be placed on a firm, evenly-supported base and specially-made aquarium stands and base units are available from aquarium dealers. Any unevenness in this base support can be eliminated by standing the tank on polystyrene sheeting or ceiling tiles. When particularly large tanks are involved, and especially when the tank is to be situated in an upstairs location, it may be necessary to check the floor supports with a local builder.

Size of aquarium

Fish can be kept in a variety of aquaria in the home, from the now infamous goldfish bowl to a several hundred gallon showpiece aquarium. The availability of a wide range of aquaria from pet and aquarium shops means that home-made tanks are largely a thing of the past. If fish are to be kept in a bowl (such as those frequently used for goldfish) a large, wide-necked bowl is preferred to the familiar glass globe, since the former permits better gaseous exchange with the atmosphere. Overall, some kind of tank is, however, recommended. Although more expensive to purchase and set up, a larger aquarium will be less prone to overstocking and fluctuations in temperature and water quality, and only slightly more expensive to maintain; in addition, it will be more interesting and attractive to look at. For a heated freshwater tank containing a range of familiar tropical (community) species, a 12-gallon (54 litre) tank should be looked upon as a minimum, with a 20-gallon (90 litres) tank the smallest tank recommended for marine fishkeeping. Tall, narrow (front to back) tanks may look more decorative when set up, but they have a smaller water surface area to volume ratio than lower, wider tanks. As a guide, home aquaria are usually between 12" (60cms) and 18" (90 cms) tall.

Equipment

When setting up an aquarium a wide range of equipment is available for the purposes of temperature control (usually heating), water circulation, aeration and filtration, and lighting. Various other pieces of minor apparatus will also be employed as part of routine tank maintenance (and these are fully described in most good aquarium books).

TYPES OF EQUIPMENT

Heating

Although not required for most coldwater species, aquarium heater-thermostats are available to maintain a steady temperature of around 73-79°F (23-26°C) in tropical freshwater and marine aquaria. As a rough guide, 5-10 watts per gallon are allowed, the lower figure for an aquarium in a heated room and the upper figure for an aquarium in an unheated room. Where possible it is advisable to use two smaller heater-thermostats rather than a single large one, since not only will this allow better heat distribution and a more even temperature, but it also reduces the risk of a complete failure of the heating system.

Heater-thermostats should be sited in a near-horizontal position usually on the rear pane of the aquarium and, if possible, in the flow of the filter and/or air stone (to assist even heat distribution). Even with the use of a reliable heater-thermostat it is important to routinely check the water temperature using an aquarium thermometer.

Filtration and aeration

Very small coldwater aquaria (including goldfish bowls) are not usually aerated or filtered, and this does not usually present any problems so long as they are not over-stocked. It is common practice to install some form of mechanical and biological filtration and aeration in larger aquaria. Details of these methods can be found in most good aquarium books, but the commonly used types of filters include:

1) Foam cartridge filters, where the water is drawn through a foam cartridge using the air from an aquarium air pump;

2) Under-gravel filters, where the air from an aquarium air pump draws the water through a 2" or 3" layer of coarse aquarium gravel (or similar substrate) situated above a filter plate on the tank floor;

3) Power filters, where different models can be situated inside or outside of the aquarium and which utilise small water pumps to pull water through a filter body containing a foam cartridge, gravel, activated carbon and/or similar filter media. Power filter pumps (power heads) are sometimes used to draw water through under-gravel filters.

Generally speaking, under-gravel filters have wide application whereas foam cartridge filters are ideal for small aquaria and power filters best suited to large tanks. When choosing a power filter it should turn over the tank volume several times during a 24 hour period, but in order to achieve optimal performance every filter has to be regularly maintained according to manufacturer's instructions.

Aeration and good general water circulation are usually provided by the filter or filters, although it is possible to augment this by using one or more air stones supplied with air from a good quality aquarium air pump. Aeration is important not only to encourage oxygen uptake by the water, but also to drive off excess carbon dioxide.

Marine aquaria, as a result of their requirement for very stable water conditions, usually rely heavily upon a number of water treatment processes or filters used in combination. Under-gravel filtration (often using a power head mounted on the uplift tube instead of an air pump and air stone), additional power filtration using an external power filter containing activated carbon, and/or protein skimming are commonly employed as may be (although less commonly) ozone and/or ultraviolet irradiation. To maintain a high degree of dissolved oxygen in the salt water of a marine and also a brackish water aquarium, additional aeration is supplied usually via an aquarium air pump and air stones. A similar overall approach can be employed for the maintenance of temperate marine organisms too. Off the shelf filtration systems are available from aquatic dealers where various components can be combined to suit the needs of individual marine aquaria. However, the importance of filter maintenance, as mentioned above, assumes paramount importance in marine tanks.

As a general guide most of the commonly employed filters and aeration devices should be used continuously, since an interruption can cause immediate and/or long-term fluctuations in water quality (especially dissolved oxygen, ammonia and nitrite levels). Nonetheless, as indicated in specialist texts, devices such as protein skimming, carbon filtration and the application of ozone can be used in a more intermittent fashion with no ill effects.

Lighting

Lighting is important in the aquarium to permit adequate viewing of the fish and to encourage healthy plant growth (if live plants are present). In marine aquaria lighting is most important for the maintenance of decorative marine algae as well as some marine invertebrates (the latter of which may contain tiny symbiotic algal cells or zooxanthellae).

Fluorescent tubes may be adequate under many circumstances. However, for the healthy maintenance of living plants in freshwater aquaria, and many algae and invertebrates such as anenomes and corals in a marine aquaria, the following lighting arrangements are recommended:

1. Freshwater aquaria with plants:

   Tanks up to 18" deep: 15-20 watts of cool white fluorescent tube lighting or 30-40 watts of tungsten bulb lighting or *Grolux* lighting per square foot of water surface.

   Tanks over 18" deep: 20-40 watts of mercury vapour or metal halide lighting per square foot of water surface.

2. Marine aquaria containing invertebrates and macro-algae:

   40-60 watts of mercury vapour or metal halide lighting per square foot of water surface. Very small tanks will, however, require less light than this.

From the above it should be apparent that tungsten bulb lighting and/or fluorescent tube lighting is adequate for shallow freshwater aquaria; in deeper fresh water tanks, and in aquaria containing many tropical marine invertebrates and macro-algae, much more intense lighting (like mercury vapour or metal halide lamps) is required. However, this type of lamp, as well as tungsten bulb lighting, does produce much more heat than fluorescent tubes and hence good water circulation is essential to prevent a build-up of heat at the water surface.

Actinic 03 tubes are recommended by some marine specialists, to be used in conjunction with metal halide lamps, to encourage tropical marine invertebrates.It is important to remember that for optimal effects fluorescent (and *Actinic*) tubes, as well as mercury vapour bulbs and metal halide burners, all have a limited effective life span and should be renewed every six to twelve months, or as recommended by their manufacturers.

To simulate tropical conditions the aquarium lights should be left on for 12 to 14 hours per day although this is probably less important in fish-only tanks.

STOCKING AQUARIA

Plants in freshwater aquaria

Live plants perform a number of useful functions in the aquarium. They provide cover for shy fish and are used by some fish to lay their eggs amongst. Some fish enjoy feeding on plants and, of course, plants are very decorative. Most importantly, plants help to maintain a natural balance in the aquarium by competing with, and helping to control, unsightly algae. As a result of the process of photosynthesis, plants also produce life-giving oxygen and use up potentially poisonous carbon dioxide during the daylight hours.

In order to grow properly it is important to ensure that plants are provided with adequate illumination (as was mentioned above). Natural sunlight is appreciated by most aquarium plants although it is a rather unpredictable (and therefore unreliable) phenomenon in temperate climates. Therefore, for good plant growth some form of artificial lighting is more or less essential.

Correct planting is also important; a mixture of garden soil and aquarium peat below the gravel on the tank floor form a good compost for most plants, although this cannot be used if under-gravel filtration is in place. Some authorities claim that under-gravel filtration can adversely affect plant growth and hence if this method of filtration is contemplated, plants are best planted in shallow trays containing a soil-peat mixture, and these can then be buried in the gravel bed. Many aquarium shops now sell a range of composts and liquid and tablet plant foods which can all be used to enhance aquarium plant growth.

It should also be kept in mind that just as with fish, certain plants prefer certain water quality parameters (especially temperature, pH and water hardness), and over-vigorous aeration may drive off too much of the in-tank carbon dioxide which would otherwise be used as a food by the plants. In fact, special aquarium carbon dioxide diffusers are now available, although these must be used in strict accordance with the manufacturers' instructions, and particular care exercised in soft, acid water where dangerous pH shifts can occur.

The very act of planting can affect plant survival and growth. Roots are best trimmed rather than bent and squashed into the gravel, and lead planting weights lightly attached to the planting roots which will help to keep the plants firmly anchored in the tank substrate.

Tall and/or bushy plants are best suited for the middle, side and rear regions of the aquarium, whilst smaller plants are ideal for the foreground region.

Coldwater fish and some (especially larger) tropical freshwater fish can be a little destructive towards live plants and hence plastic plants are a decorative alternative.

Tank decor

A huge range of items can be used as tank decor. As a general rule anything that is purchased from an aquarium shop should be safe to use. Avoid most metals (lead weights are safe), limestone and chalk rocks in most freshwater aquaria (since these can cause the pH and water hardness to rise to an unacceptable level), and green woods (which can rot and release undesirable substances into the water).

Bogwood is a particular type of decorative wood that is sold by many aquarium shops. Used in an untreated fashion, it may add a brown colouration to the water, although this can be prevented by boiling the wood two or three times and/or completely enclosing it within two or three coats of exterior quality polyurathane varnish.

If in doubt about any item of decor, its suitability can be established by placing it in a bucket of tank water with several inexpensive fish for a week or so.

Fish and invertebrates

The choice of livestock for the freshwater and marine aquarium is large, although guidance on choice, suitability and compatibility can be obtained from any good aquarium dealer or an aquarium textbook. Water quality preferences (especially temperature, pH and water hardness in freshwater aquaria), the social requirements of the species (whether it is to be kept as a lone individual, as a pair or as a small shoal), and its compatibility with other fish and/or invertebrate species and plants are all factors to be considered. Similarly, fish disease treatments are toxic to a number ·of invertebrates, which can cause difficulties when fish and invertebrates are kept together in the same aquarium.

An indication of the maximum recommended stocking levels for fish are provided in the checklist of appendix 2. These levels may be exceeded by experienced hobbyists in mature aquaria, but should be built-up gradually over several weeks or even months in new aquaria. The addition of too many fish, too soon, will over-load the initial capacity of the filtration system of a new tank perhaps resulting in high levels of nitrite and ammonia and even cause fish deaths. This "new tank syndrome" can be avoided by adding just small numbers of fish over a protracted period, by routinely checking nitrite and ammonia levels, by carrying out larger than usual partial water changes as required, and by checking filter maintenance. Stocking levels for marine invertebrates are less restrictive, although it is important to take account of the interactions which can occur between fish and invertebrates and even between invertebrates. The quarantine of new fish is mentioned in Chapter 22. Whenever new fish are brought home they should be floated in their polythene bag in the tank for fifteen to twenty minutes to let the temperatures equalise and then the tank and transport water should be gradually mixed before releasing the fish completely. Turning off the tank lights and/or feeding the other fish in the tank can all help the new fish to settle-in.

MAINTENANCE

Full details of recommended tank maintenance can be found in most good aquarium books. Here the importance of careful feeding, regular partial water changes and proper filter maintenance will be emphasised.

Feeding

Overfeeding is extremely common and a major source of problems amongst new hobbyists. As a rough guide fish should be fed two to four times per day with only as much food as is eaten in a few minutes. A good quality flaked, pellet or tablet food with the occasional use of frozen, freeze-dried or live foods (all available from aquarium shops) is all that is required for the vast majority of aquarium fish. The accumulation of uneaten food will precipitate problems including high levels of nitrite and ammonia, and excessive algal growths, and must be avoided.

The fact that most fish can go two or even three weeks with little or no food makes the holiday care of fish very simple, and the use of aquarium vacation food blocks is largely redundant.

Partial Water Changes

In addition to careful feeding, regular partial water changes are also important as part of routine tank care. Every two to four weeks or so about 25% of the tank volume be discarded and replaced with dechlorinated tap water of similar quality. A simple siphon tube or a gravel washer (available from an aquarium shop) means that the tank substrate can be cleaned as part of the water change. Larger, more infrequent water changes will bring about less desirable fluctuations in water conditions, which can have adverse effects on sensitive species, especially some marine fish and invertebrates.

Filter Maintenance

With the water levels in the tank lowered as a result of a partial water change, this is a good opportunity to attend to filter maintenance. A siphon tube or gravel washer can be used to great effect in a tank which relies on under-gravel filtration as it prevents a build-up of debris in the gravel bed with consequent clogging and loss of filter efficiency. Other filter media will also require regular cleaning or replacement in order to maintain water conditions, and a gradual reduction in water output from the filter and/or the onset of water quality and even disease problems may indicate the need for more attention to filter maintenance. Most filters contain rich bacterial flora which is responsible for nitrification (the aerobic conversion of ammonia to nitrite to nitrate), hence complete or even large-scale replacement of the medium or media in a filter can precipitate a rise in nitrite or ammonia levels until the bacterial flora becomes re-established. However, gentle rinsing of (for example) foam cartridges (a common filter medium) in lukewarm water on a fortnightly or monthly basis does not usually affect nitrification to an unacceptable extent. Other filter media usually come with recommendations concerning their renewal or replacement.

CHAPTER FOUR

POND FISHKEEPING

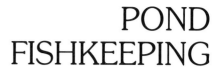

Chris Andrews

TYPES OF PONDKEEPING

The majority of garden ponds contain a range of coldwater fish species notably goldfish, carp, koi carp, tench and orfe, and are often relatively well-planted. Accessories and equipment are usually kept to a minimum and the establishment of local wildlife (e.g. aquatic insects and amphibians) in the pond may be encouraged. However, the establishment of ponds especially for the maintenance of koi carp, usually with a minimum of submerged vegetation and sometimes with quite elaborate filtration systems, is increasing.

IMPORTANT CONSIDERATIONS

Pond construction

There are three basic methods of pond construction: concrete, moulded glass fibre, and plastic or polythene flexible liners. The construction of a garden pond from concrete is hard work and although the finished article is permanent, it may crack as a result of frost and ice. Moulded pools are very easy to install but can be expensive and some are too shallow (see below) to maintain fish through the coldest winter months.

Flexible liners are a popular choice; several types exist ranging from little more than a thin sheet of plastic or polythene, to very tough butyl liners which are almost as permanent as a concrete or moulded pool. Full details on pond construction can be found in the popular literature.

Siting a pond

A garden pond is best situated in an area of level ground where it receives some shade from the mid-afternoon summer sunshine and some protection from the cold winter winds. Nonetheless, it should not be sited below over-hanging trees and bushes (which may shed their leaves into the pool in the autumn, causing pollution), and the entry of fertilised or pesticide run-off into the pool should also be prevented.

Naturally, a tapwater supply will be needed to fill the pond, top-up evaporative losses and carry out occasional water changes, with any excess water being discarded to the surrounding garden or to a soakaway. Fountain pumps, filters, pond heaters and pond lights all require a source of electrical power, provided according to the equipment manufacturers' safety instructions.

Size of ponds

A pond may be almost any size and shape although it should always have an area deeper than 18" (90 cms), to provide protection for the fish during the colder months and some shallow shelves for emergent vegetation and perhaps fish spawning. Generally speaking garden ponds are always longer and wider than they are deep (to provide a reasonable water surface area), and 6 ft. (approx. 2m) long, by 4 ft. (approx.1.5m) wide, by up to 1.5 ft. (approx. 0.9m) deep is suggested as a minimum size. Very small ponds will be prone to overstocking and fluctuating water conditions.

Equipment

A number of items of optional equipment are frequently used by pond keepers.

Small water pump fountain units add attractive water movement to the pond, as well as providing aeration in warm, still weather. Such pumps can also be used to provide water for a waterfall and some can be converted to also carry out a small amount of mechanical and/or biological filtration. More elaborate filters are available and are commonly used in association with koi keeping. Such filters can result in very clear water as well as encouraging very stable water quality conditions. Under-gravel filters over some or all of the pond bottom are used, although it is more common to -treated use some form of out-of-pond system which may range from a single polythene water tank filled with gravel, to compartmental concrete filter tanks, high-pressure sand filters and even ultraviolet irradiation. Naturally, such systems require a pump to pass water through the filter tank or tanks (usually at least several times during a twenty-four hour period) and regular filter maintenance is essential for their efficient running.

As was mentioned above, for indoor aquaria, the aeration and filtration devices for garden ponds must not be turned off for long periods during the spring/summer although it is common practice to turn them off (or at least reduce their flows) each winter and turn them on (or up) again the following early spring.

Low wattage electrical pond heaters are available and can be used to keep a small area of the pond surface free from ice during a hard winter, thus permitting continued gaseous exchange with the atmosphere. Such heaters do not warm the water enough to affect fish activity.

Although irrelevant to the fish and plants in a garden pond, decorative lighting units are available to illuminate the pond and the surround area.

STOCKING PONDS

Plants

As was described for freshwater aquaria, plants can carry out a number of very important functions and their effect on algal growth and on stabilising water conditions are both particularly pertinent in garden ponds.

The simplest and most convenient way to plant out a pond is using the baskets that are available from most retail outlets. These come in a range of sizes and permit easy rearrangement of plants at a later date. The baskets are best lined with clean sacking and then filled with unfertilised garden soil. Following careful planting of these baskets, and before placing them into the pond, a layer of pea gravel or pebbles can be added to the basket to prevent fish disturbing the soil causing discolouration of the water.

Pond plants are generally divided into marginals, deep water aquatics, floating plants and lilies. Full details on pond plants and their preference (especially with regard to water depth) can be found in most good pond books.

Fish

A smaller range of fish are generally kept in a garden pond than in an indoor aquarium and these fish are often limited to specifically ornamental varieties that are brightly coloured and easily visible. Some of the more unusual and long-finned varieties of goldfish are, however, a little delicate to be left in the pond throughout the year and may develop fin problems in cool weather. Other types of fish such as those native to the UK, Europe and North America may be kept in a garden pond but are less distinctively marked and therefore less easily seen and appreciated. Salmonoid fish such as trout do not usually fare particularly well in a garden pond, where temperatures may get too high and dissolved oxygen levels too low. Naturally predatory species (pike, perch and coldwater catfish) should be avoided they will be rarely seen and will grow and feed on the other fish. Certain species of tropical freshwater fish can be kept in a garden pond during the warmer months.

Invertebrates and Amphibians

Various invertebrates (e.g. snails, crayfish) can be added to the pond but are of questionable benefit, and (in the case of crayfish) will be seldom seen. Amphibians can co-exist quite well, although the fish may eat some of the amphibian young and amorous male frogs and toads are a potential, although seldom-realised hazard, as they grab at passing fish during their spring breeding season.

Stocking levels

An indication of the maximum safe stocking level for fish in a garden pond is provided in the checklist of appendix 2. Although this may be exceeded by experienced pond keepers, especially if some form of filtration or aeration is used, it is a useful guide for a newly-established pond as it includes a margin for fish growth. Stocking should begin with a number of relatively inexpensive fish (to ensure there are no unforeseen problems) and then proceed towards the above-maximum figure over a few weeks. "New pond syndrome" (as opposed to "new tank syndrome") is less often referred to in the hobbyist literature, although it is still unwise to stock a pond with too many fish too soon.

Quarantine

Since infectious diseases can be quite difficult to treat in a large garden pond, quarantine of all new fish is quite important (see Chapter 22). All new fish should be floated in their new home or in the quarantine tank for fifteen to twenty minutes, to let water temperatures equalise.

POND MAINTENANCE AND SEASONAL EFFECTS

Situated in an outdoor environment, seasonal changes (especially with regard to temperature) have a major influence on pond maintenance. This is referred to in detail in most good books on pond keeping, but the major considerations are given below.

Feeding

As water temperatures fall below 54°F (12°C), the appetite of most pond fish will decrease, and below 46-50°F (8° or 10°C) most pond fish will cease feeding altogether and become dormant. As a result, extra care must be exercised to avoid overfeeding in cool weather, and feeding suspended for most of the winter. If the fish are active on a warm day in winter, small feeds will do them no harm. Uneaten food must never be allowed to accumulate in the pond however. As a rough guide during the spring/summer, pond fish should be fed two to four times a day on a good quality flake, pellet or stick foods, offering only enough that can be consumed in a few minutes.

Plant growth

Plant growth will increase through the spring and summer with an autumn die-back, when all the dead and dying plant material should be removed from the pond. A coarse-meshed net over the pond will prevent autumn leaves entering and rotting in the pond which can result in pollution problems.

Algal blooms

These are caused by tiny suspended algal cells causing green water, or beds of filamentous algae. They can be both unsightly and potentially dangerous for the fish. Like plants, the algae photosynthesise during the day so there is a nett output of oxygen, although this ceases overnight when there may be a nett uptake of oxygen as the algal material carries on respiring. In addition, the sudden die-back of an algal bloom can result in large amounts of rotting material in the pond and obvious pollution problems. Algal blooms are normally caused by a number of factors including too much sunlight, too few submerged plants, inadequate shading, over-feeding of the fish and fertilised run-off from the garden entering the pond after heavy rain. Algal treatments are available from most good aquatic shops, but these should be used with care as they may bring about a massive algal die-back and consequent problems. The prevention and treatment of algal blooms in garden ponds is dealt with in most good pond books.

Pond disturbance

This should be kept to a minimum during the cooler months of the year, with one or two partial water changes carried out during the summer and early autumn. Should the pond ice over during the winter, a small hole should be melted in the ice using boiling water thus permitting gaseous exchange with the atmosphere. A pool heater will prevent this icing up, and the ice must never be smashed with a hammer or rock as the shock waves may harm the fish. New fish and plants are best added in the spring and summer when they have plenty of time to settle in before the winter. Every few years a major overhaul may be required; this should be carried out in the early summer before the plants begin growing in earnest. The winter care and maintenance of filters was mentioned above.

CHAPTER FIVE

NUTRITION

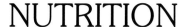

David M Ford

GENERAL CONSIDERATIONS

Fish have the same catabolic energy processes as warm-blooded mammals, hence their basic nutritional requirements are similar. Differences in physiology, however, do mean there are some special considerations. Dietary energy is utilised mainly for body maintenance, growth and reproduction, little or no energy being required to maintain body temperature or the fish's position in the water.

There are also wide species differences in nutritional requirements reflected in their carnivorous/ herbivorous habit and differences in the anatomy and physiology of their digestive tract (see Chapter 1).

NUTRITIONAL REQUIREMENTS

Proteins

In the wild, carnivorous or omnivorous fish eat a high protein diet. Farmed edible fish are also fed a high protein diet to maximise growth rates for commercial reasons. This can lead to the amino acids being utilised as an energy source as well as for growth, with the resultant production of ammonia. High water flow systems used in farming flush this away, but this is impractical in the home aquarium or pond.

To avoid this rise in ammonia, a high quality protein source should be used so that lower levels are nutritionally effective. Trials at the Waltham Centre for Pet Nutrition showed that 30 to 35% digestible protein is sufficient for ornamental fish. The energy sources are then taken from the carbohydrate content of the food which breaks down to non-polluting carbon dioxide and water. This is obviously very important for maintaining good water quality (see Chapter 2).

The proportion of particular amino acids in the protein is also an important factor - lysine and methionine being at particularly high levels in fish flesh. Specific clinical signs have been attributed to deficiencies of certain essential amino acids (see Chapter 15).

Fats

Since fish are poikilothermic they cannot regulate their body temperature. The highest temperature the average pet fish will experience is about 25°C in the central heated home, or the thermostatically controlled tropical aquarium. Fish therefore store fat as unsaturated oils, since the saturated fats of the higher animals would be solid at these low body temperatures. For this reason, traditional human foods are unsuitable for fish to eat. Fat-containing foods such as hamburgers, sausages and formed-meat chunks can actually block the gut of fish with solid fat.

Meat-based pet foods are unsuitable for the same reason. Fish based foods are more suitable, but the vitamin content may be comparatively low after processing. Similarly, land-based vegetables are not very suitable for feeding to herbivorous fish since their natural diet consists mainly of algae.

Vitamins and Minerals

The correct balance of vitamins (including Vit. C) and minerals is essential, although there may be species variations in the exact requirements. In processed foods vitamins may be destroyed, so this needs to be allowed for during the manufacturing process. The vitamin and mineral needs may also be increased during periods of stress, and so extra supplements may be useful at such times. A discussion of the deficiency induced diseases is given in Chapter 15.

TYPES OF FOOD

Live Foods

Logically the best diet for fish would be the same as that in the wild, i.e. mainly living animals or plants. The problem with reproducing this living diet in the home aquarium is that of parasites. Over millions of years parasites have used the food chain to infest fish in a balanced way that ensures survival of parasite and carrier. In the confines of the home aquarium the balance is tipped towards the parasite and agents such as *Ichthyophthirius*, *Lernia*, *Chilodonella*, *Camallanus* and so on, will multiply until the fish dies. Hence the common source of these parasites, live aquatic foods, must not be added to the aquarium or even the pond. Daphnia and Tubifex worms are sold as the ideal live food, but microscopic examination of these foods will usually reveal parasites either within the body of the animal or swimming with them. The same comment applies to all the other live foods from blood worms to larvae.

It is possible to cultivate some of these animals, isolating them from sources of infestation. A good example is the hatching of brine shrimp eggs for first-feeding to fry. However, where live food is required, for example, to condition the fish for breeding, it is best to use non-aquatic live food (e.g. the garden earthworm, aphids from unsprayed roses, small land snails, slugs and flies). None will carry aquatic parasites. Cultured live foods are also available (e.g. white worms, micro worms and fruit flies).

Commercial Diets

The most convenient foods are the commercially produced flake foods or pellets. The flakes consist of tiny plates of blended raw materials that are dried to under 4% moisture level to prevent bacterial or fungal growth, hence improving shelf life. They not only provide the fish with the correct nutrient requirements, but are also free from the hazards of introducing disease.

Larger fish such as Oscars, *Astronotus ocellatus*, will find flake food too small. However, they still need the necessary vitamins and minerals that commercial foods contain. This problem can be overcome by inserting a couple of flakes into slits made in the chunks of fish flesh that are normally fed.

Quantity to feed

Fish have an ability to eat continuously, digest what they need and excrete the rest. The common goldfish has been called the underwater cow, and its continuous searching for food encourages the owner to overfeed, and hence pollute the aquarium .

Trials by Professor Klontz of the University of Idaho, USA, using 'Aquarian' Flake Food have revealed that growing ornamental fish require 5% of body weight in 3 or more feeds daily. Survival alone requires 1% of body weight. In flake terms this means an average Tropical Community fish (such as the Serpae Tetra, *Hyphessobrycon serpae*) weighing 0.5 gm needs 0.025 gm or 3 flakes (20 mm) daily, either all at once, or preferably divided into 3 feeds per day.

Obviously, declaring feed weights is not practical, and so manufacturers usually recommend to feed sparingly, i.e. enough to give 2 or 3 minutes of continuous feeding per day. Generally, after ingesting a few flakes the fish's gut is full and the fish swims away from the feeding area. The surplus flake should then be removed.

CHAPTER SIX

THE FISH TRADE

David M Ford

The most popular fish (indeed most popular pet) is the common goldfish, and these fish are mass produced in fish farms throughout the World, from China (where the fish originated) to the UK.

Tropical fish are the next most popular, and these originate in the World's tropics from the Amazon jungles of South America to an Indian river or a Thailand lake. Most are now mass produced in commercial fish farms in the tropical areas. A classic example is the Neon Tetra, *Paracheirodon innesi*. The fish originates from tributaries of the Amazon, but many years ago breeding pairs were taken to the Hong Kong fish farms where they are now bred in millions to satisfy the world demand. In fact fish listings now call the *Paracheirodon innesi* the 'Hong Kong Tetra'.

Marine fishkeeping is a small, but keen section of the hobby. The beautiful Coral fish are kept in synthetic seawater, with continuous biological filtration. These fish have not yet been successfully farmed, therefore all the fish in the trade are wild caught. At one time dynamite and solutions of Cyanide were used in the coral reefs to stun or anaesthetise the fish. These malpractices have now ceased and only hand caught specimens are available, making them very expensive.

The most expensive fish in the trade are the Japanese Koi Carp. Each variety of these large pond fish has a special Japanese name to describe the colour patterns, and prize winning specimens change hands at thousands of £'s each.

The Size of Trade

The last survey of the World market in Tropical fish was back in 1975 when the Food & Agricultural Organisation of the United Nations sponsored a study (FAO Circular No. 335) that revealed the total value of the trade was 4,000,000 USA Dollars. This must have doubled over the decade or so since then, which makes it a valuable foreign currency earner for the Far Eastern countries.

The main importers are U.S.A and Europe . In the UK, 2 million households own ornamental fish, whereas the figure is nearly 20 million in the U.S.A. In numbers of fish per head of population, Germany is the leader.

The Import Trade

There is a mass movement of farmed fish from the tropics to the temperate zones. The majority are flown out from major airports, such as Singapore, Hong Kong and Kuala Lumpur to London, New York and Frankfurt. It is estimated that several hundred million fish are being flown around the World annually. An estimate of the sources of World ornamental fish is:

Eastern Asia	69% mainly Tropicals
Latin America	27% Tropicals
Africa	2% Tropicals (Cichlids)
Japan	1.5% Koi and Goldfish

The Asian fish originate from Hong Kong (23%), Singapore (12%), Thailand (6%), Taiwan (6%), Phillipines (6%), Indonesia (2%), as well as India, Sri Lanka and Malaysia.

Wild Fish

There are still some wild caught species supplied to the trade, especially those fish that give problems in captive breeding, such as Scats (*Scatophagidae*) and Spiny Eels (*Mastocembelidae*) and, of course, all the Marines. Some species are wild caught because the local people have not the will or the facilities to set-up farms (e.g. Brazil and Central Africa).

All exported fish from Brazil are wild specimens with between 10 and 20 million fish being caught in the Amazon basin (FAO of UN Co-operation Programme Report on Brazil 1978). 85% of these fish are Cardinal Tetras (*Cheirodon axelrodi*) and 6% are Corydoras (mostly *Corydoras julii*). The remainder are mainly Discus (*Symphysodon*) and Bleeding Heart Tetras (*Hyphesrubrostigma*).

Although wild caught fish are often larger and sometimes more colourful than their farmed cousins, they always suffer from parasites and often carry diseases. Few UK Importers will order fish direct from South America because of these problems, preferring to buy quarantined fish from suppliers in Germany.

African fish are mainly Rift Valley Cichlids, but these are one group of fish that have been successfully bred by local breeders rather than commercial fish farms. Many of the specimens in the trade can be traced back to enthusiasts who studied and then bred the fish, such as the British Cichlid Association members. A few expatriate collectors live in Africa and ship wild fish mainly via Nigeria.

American Fish Farms

Florida is the home of the USA ornamental fish farming industry. The unusual climate of the area means that frequent rain storms soak into the land (it was an ancient coral reef) and the water can be tapped and pumped into concrete ponds at a constant 70°F. The sun soon raises the temperature to 80°F for mass breeding of most Tropical fish.

These farmers are very efficient and produce good quality fish with little labour, so the costs are not much greater than the Far Eastern Fish Farms with their plentiful cheap labour and no temperature problems. The Americans use a sub-contract system, where large units produce breeding stock for smaller farms and buy back the fish they produce. These sub-contractors use aquariums rather than ponds, so Florida is now the source of the best tank reared popular Tropicals such as Harlequins, Clown Loaches, most Cichlids and Killifish. UK Importers are increasingly ordering USA fish, flown direct from Miami to London.

Far East Farms

Hong Kong, Thailand, Singapore and Malaysia have numerous fish farms in the jungles surrounding their main cities. Some are simply netted areas in local streams so that local fish can breed without natural predation. Most are concrete ponds with palm leaf rooves to shade the water from the midday sun.

The more sophisticated farms breed just one species of fish, and may develop special varieties or 'sports' (e.g. Veiltail Angels or Albino Catfish).

Aquatic plants may be produced by bubbling carbon dioxide from cylinders into loam based shallow ponds. They are harvested and shrink wrapped onto polythene trays for export.

The exporter's HQ is based near the airport where there are facilities to bag the fish, flush the bag with pure oxygen and then pack them in polystyrene boxes to maintain temperature. The shipments are containerised with other perishables such as fruits, flowers and vegetables. Standards are maintained by Government Inspectors or Veterinarians, and each shipment will carry the necessary certification.

The UK Importer

The main expense in importing live fish is the airfreight cost of the water. For small orders, individual aquarium shops may buy from a wholesale importer, or become part of a consortium. This involves all the local aquarium shops combining their order so one large shipment is placed with a shipping agent. The minimum shipment is 100 kilos, which is 10 or 12 polystyrene boxes of water filled polybags. The number of fish in that shipment varies enormously because the polybag may contain just one giant catfish, or 2000 neons. Wholesalers can place orders large enough not to need a consortium, but consolidation of orders may still be made by the shipping agent. For example, a regular Monday arrival at Manchester Airport from Singapore is the B747 Combi containing some 400 boxes of live tropical fishes, which represents orders from wholesalers or consortiums around the country, consolidated by the shipping agent for the minimum shipping costs.

The principal traders of this industry are part of OFI, Ornamental Fish International. This universal self-regulatory body ensures the fish are properly looked after in their flights, and everyone from the jungle farmer to the high street retailer gets a fair deal.

CHAPTER SEVEN

ENVIRONMENTAL ASPECTS

Edward J Branson

Peter J Southgate

GENERAL CONSIDERATIONS

Healthy fish are in equilibrium with their environment and any disease organisms present in that environment. Changes in environmental conditions can upset this balance and influence the development of disease in a number of ways:

1. A direct toxic effect of the environmental parameter (e.g: High levels of ammonia producing gill disease).

2. An indirect effect by altering the toxicity of other environmental parameters (e.g: a low pH reducing ammonia toxicity).

3. An indirect effect by causing stress which subsequently reduces the fish's resistance to disease from other sources.

The objective in any fish holding system is therefore to create and maintain good water quality and, probably just as important, to maintain a stable environment.

The environmental aspects influencing fish health and disease can be broadly classified into the following groups:

1. Dissolved gases (oxygen, nitrogen, carbon dioxide, ammonia, hydrogen sulphide,and methane).
2. Miscellaneous water quality parameters (pH, hardness, conductivity, temperature, and suspended solids).
3. Metabolic waste products.
4. Exogenous materials.

DISSOLVED GASES

Oxygen

Deficiency - Oxygen is the most important of the dissolved gases and adequate levels must be maintained. Typical symptoms of oxygen deficiency are 'gasping' at the surface and gathering at water inlets. This can be caused by oxygen deficiency in the water, gill damage, which will impair oxygen uptake, and anaemia, which reduces oxygen bio-availability. In situations with marginal oxygen levels, signs of oxygen deficiency often appear after feeding or at times of high stress when the oxygen demand is greatest.

Oxygen deficiency can arise from inadequate oxygenation. Water at high temperatures or high salinities will hold less oxygen than equivalent bodies of cooler fresh water. De-oxygenation can result from a large biological oxygen demand (BOD). This can happen typically when large amounts of organic matter are being degraded aerobically. A further factor is the respiratory requirements of large quantities of water plants which can cause de-oxygenation overnight, producing symptoms in the early morning before photosynthesis re-oxygenates the water.

Algal blooms in ponds are usually seen in the spring, when water nutrient levels are high due to the winter degradation of dead plants. They occur as soon as there is sufficient warmth and light for the algae to grow. These blooms can typically produce de-oxygenation during the night and, to a certain extent, clogging of gills. Once the algae have used up the available nutrients they will die back creating a large BOD, again potentially causing de-oxygenation. Blooms can also occur to a lesser extent in the autumn, feeding on nutrients released by the decay of the spring algae and other water plants. Thus it should be ensured that adequate oxygenation is maintained, and that there is no build up of dead organic matter.

Some algae can produce direct toxicity causing tissue damage, typically in the gill and liver.

Supersaturation with oxygen can occur, usually associated with algal bloom oxygen production, but this problem is more commonly associated with nitrogen.

Nitrogen

Supersaturation - Supersaturation with nitrogen is usually due to faulty pumps sucking in air under pressure, but can also occur when saturated water is heated, thus reducing the solubility of the gas, prior to adding it to aquaria. The condition produced is similar to the bends seen in divers, with gas bubbles forming within blood vessels and manifesting themselves as '**gas bubble disease**'. Small bubbles form in superficial blood vessels and can be seen, typically, on gills and fins, and also behind the eye. If supersaturation is present, it can usually be detected by placing an object in the water, when many small bubbles will immediately form on it. The problem can be cured within the system by agitation, or just aerating inflowing water in order to allow excess gas to escape. Nothing can be done to treat individual fish, and those that recover will often be runts and/or more susceptible to disease. A chronic form of this disease can occur due to low level supersaturation, and this can result in cataracts, fin rot and gill disease.

Carbon Dioxide

Carbon dioxide can cause problems if present at high levels. This will tend to occur at an acid pH due to the dissociation reaction of the gas in water. High levels can interfere with oxygen uptake, and can also cause **nephrocalcinosis**, where calcium carbonate is deposited within the kidney tubules. There is no treatment for this latter condition.

Ammonia, Hydrogen sulphide, and Methane

Ammonia is produced as a direct result of the metabolism of the fish and from the decomposition of organic matter. Hydrogen sulphide and Methane are products of the anaerobic breakdown of organic matter, and are directly toxic causing rapid death with few, if any, diagnostic signs. Unexplained deaths following pond or tank cleaning can often be explained by the release of these gasses from sediments.

METABOLIC WASTE PRODUCTS

The most important of these are ammonia and nitrites, the former being probably the second most important water quality parameter after dissolved oxygen.

Ammonia

Un-ionised ammonia will primarily cause direct gill epithelial damage with consequent hyperplasia and reduced ability to take up oxygen. Depending on the species, there may also be liver, kidney and brain damage with reduced activity and growth. The level of un-ionised ammonia will vary with the pH and temperature, it being minimised by low values of both these parameters (see chapter 2).

Nitrites

Nitrites are highly toxic to fish, and if present at sufficient levels can cause the production of methaemoglobin, with consequent hypoxia and cyanosis.

Faecal material

This can be significant because, along with waste food, it can contribute to de-oxygenation if it is degraded aerobically, and can give rise to methane and hydrogen sulphide if degraded by anaerobic bacteria. In addition, faecal material will contribute to organic suspended solids which can cause gill problems.

MISCELLANEOUS WATER QUALITY PARAMETERS

pH

This is related directly to the hardness/alkalinity/buffering capacity of the water. It should be maintained within tolerable limits for the species in question, and should not be allowed to vary significantly or stress related problems may ensue. Generally the optimum pH range for most species is between pH 6 and pH 9, and outside this range direct toxic effects can occur, and stress levels will be high.

In alkaline water effects vary, but generally with a pH greater than 10 most species will die, and those that survive will usually suffer gill damage and changes to the lens and cornea producing opacity. These sub-lethal effects may be seen with a pH greater than 9 in some species.

With acidic water, rising levels of H^+ ions will cause direct gill and epidermal damage, resulting in reduced oxygen uptake and osmoregulatory problems. Generally a pH of less than 4 will kill most species, with sub-lethal effects occurring with pH values less than 5.

Problems can arise when water changes are made in aquaria. If the buffering capacity is low, then the pH will naturally fall with time due to the acidity of metabolic waste products. If water changes are then carried out using water with an appreciably higher pH than that in the tank, there will be a sudden rise in pH which will be extremely stressful to the fish. It is therefore important to ensure that buffering capacity is sufficient to prevent this.

In ponds, acid rain may have a significant effect. There may also be problems in ponds supplied by natural water courses which arise in acid areas. After rain, especially following a dry spell, acid flushes can occur in streams. Heavy metals are more soluble in acid water, and consequently heavy metal toxicity can be associated with acidity problems.

Hardness

This affects the toxicity of certain heavy metals. Generally the softer the water, the more toxic any metal that is present.

Conductivity

This is a measurement of the ion content of water, and is a potential stressor if high or fluctuating. In aquaria where evaporation losses are replaced with anything other than distilled water, there will be a tendency for the ion concentration of the water to rise. Partial water changes should prevent this from happening.

Temperature

This should ideally be kept constant, but if variations do occur, they should happen very slowly (as a rule, no more than 1°C change every 2 minutes). When fish are moved, there should not be a temperature difference of more than 2-3°C. Rapid changes can result in temperature shock and consequent stress.

Suspended solids

These are usually not a problem except in ponds supplied with water from natural water courses. In these cases, occasional flushes of suspended solids should be expected. These can cause stress and clogging of the gills, with a possible increase in the incidence of bacterial gill disease. If the material is irritant, actual gill damage may occur resulting in excessive mucus production, 'coughing' and gill hypertrophy and hyperplasia. In all cases there is a reduction in the efficiency of oxygen uptake.

Exogenous materials

This category covers all those materials, whether natural or man-made, which may be present or introduced into the water, and which are potentially harmful. They are considered in greater detail in chapter 13, but include:

1. Heavy metals from the water supply, food, or leached from equipment.
2. Chlorine from tap water used for topping up aquaria or ponds.
3. Pesticides/herbicides etc. from misuse of these chemicals or by contamination of water supplies.
4. Chemicals used for treatments.
5. Poisons from water supplies or maliciously introduced.

MISCELLANEOUS FACTORS

Many other factors can cause disturbance of the status quo, for example:

1. Sunburn - fish with no cover, in clear water and exposed to strong sunlight can suffer from sunburn.
2. Damage due to excessive handling or violent spawning behaviour.
3. Vandalism - many ornamental fish have suffered damage at the hands of brick throwing or stick wielding vandals.

(These three categories can result in skin damage which, apart from causing stress, can lead to secondary infection with bacteria or fungi. In addition skin damage can seriously impair osmoregulatory control.)

4. Overstocking - this can be extremely stressful in some species.
5. Vibration - due to local heavy traffic or, for example, explosions in the vicinity can cause severe stress.
6. Birds - birds such as herons can predate fish and also introduce parasites such as eye-fluke.
7. Other animals - snails may act as intermediate hosts for certain parasites such as eye flukes, frogs can act as a reservoir host for *Aeromonas hydrophila*.

CHAPTER EIGHT

PROTOZOAL PARASITES

Edward J Branson
Peter J Southgate

GENERAL CONSIDERATIONS

A small number of protozoa living in, or on fish should be considered normal. This harmonious host-parasite relationship can be disrupted in conditions of high stress, such as overcrowding and poor water quality, or where the host fish is debilitated or in poor health. The result is multiplication of the parasite and consequent disease.

Closed systems, such as ponds or recirculating aquaria, can allow a large build-up of parasites during a disease outbreak. Not only will weak fish then be at risk, but the level of organisms may be such that the defences of even healthy fish are overwhelmed. Thus it is important that infested fish are isolated.

Treatment of all parasitic diseases should be aimed at improving the underlying environmental conditions and health of the fish, and reduction of parasite numbers. The number of free living organisms within the aquarium or pond, may be reduced by increasing the number of water changes or the water flow rate. The use of an appropriate chemical treatment will reduce the number of parasites on the fish themselves. Gill damage, a common consequence of ectoparasitism, may make the fish very susceptible to chemical treatment, so great care must be taken when treatments are carried out.

Any chemical treatment used must take into account the life cycle of the parasite. Most of the important protozoan parasites have a direct life cycle (i.e: they do not require secondary hosts), although some of the life cycle stages may occur off the primary host.

New fish introduced into a system will almost certainly harbour a few parasites, and the stress of movement may well precipitate disease caused by these parasites. To ensure that this risk is reduced, new fish should be quarantined before introducing them to the main system. A quarantine period of 4 weeks should be adequate for most parasite problems to become apparent, as well as those caused by bacteria and viruses. The same applies to plants and rocks, which may also carry fish parasites. Prophylactic treatments may be advisable during quarantine.

Generally, protozoan parasites affect either the outside or the inside of the fish, seldom both, and for the purposes of this chapter will be divided accordingly. Taxonomic considerations will only be taken into account where relevant to diagnosis.

ECTOPARASITIC PROTOZOA

Parasite / Commensal Relationships

Protozoa which inhabit the external surfaces of fish are either true parasites or commensals. In the case of parasites, any imbalance can cause serious problems for the host. With commensals, although some tissue debris may be consumed, the organisms do not feed on healthy fish tissues, merely using the fish as a convenient feeding platform. These commensals are only likely to have an adverse effect if numbers become so large that the sheer physical mass of the animals causes a problem.

General signs

A common sign of external parasitism is 'flashing', when the fish attempts to free itself of the irritation caused by the parasite. Fish will suddenly dart across the tank or pond, often turning on their side showing their lighter underside (the flash). The movement often involves rubbing the affected part against some object in the tank, or breaking the surface of the water.

The irritation usually leads to an increase in mucus production from infested areas. This can result in localised or general grey colouration and possibly trailing strings of mucus, especially from affected gills. An increased level of mucus may cause the water to foam. This increase in mucus is the reason that many ectoparasitic diseases are known as **slime disease**. In cases of long standing, severe ectoparasitism, the mucus producing cells can become exhausted. In this case, the fish will have less mucus than normal, and may well feel 'dry' to the touch.

Lethargy and loss of appetite are common symptoms, with evidence of respiratory distress if the gills are affected. Fin clamping, where fins are held tight against the body, is often seen in species where this behaviour is abnormal. Local or general colour change may occur. Damage to skin or gills, either directly by the parasite, or due to rubbing, can lead to invasion by opportunist bacteria or fungi, which may obscure the primary aetiology.

Microscopic examination of freshly prepared gill and skin scrapes for external protozoa is described in chapter 20. It should be remembered, however, that these organisms will die quite quickly if allowed to dry out, and will also suffer from lack of oxygen. As they are most easily seen when moving, it is advisable to keep them as active as possible by ensuring that the water in which the fish are kept prior to sampling is well oxygenated. Samples should be kept moist with the water in which the fish were kept, and they should be examined as soon as possible after sampling.

Disease Organisms

The main protozoal groups associated with ectoparasitic disease, and the names of some of the diseases produced are listed opposite.

FLAGELLATES

Ichthyobo sp. (Costiasis)

Ichthyobodo sp. (previously *Costia* sp.) cause the disease **costiasis**, one of the causes of **slime disease**. They are found worldwide on freshwater fish, and have a wide temperature range. Marine species may exist, but have not been seen in aquarium fish. Fish eggs and amphibians can be affected.

Characteristics - Occurs on the host as a free swimming form, and also attached to epidermal cells. The free swimming form is oval to bean shaped, flattened and 5 to 20µm in length. From one end arise 2 flagella. One is free, the other recurrent and fixed in a groove along the body. Two pairs of flagella may be seen just before division. The attached form is pyriform in shape, does not have any visible flagella, and causes direct damage to the cell. In the right conditions, they can reproduce very rapidly, the rate depending on temperature. They are obligate parasites, with a direct life cycle spent entirely on the host. They are thought to pass from one fish to another through the water. Cysts may occur in the environment in adverse conditions.

Disease - Typical signs of external parasitism. The skin or gills may be infested, and when fins are affected they usually have a ragged appearance.

Diagnosis - Skin scrapes of affected areas show motile organisms moving with a characteristic erratic spiralling movement. Magnification of x400 may be necessary as they are approximately the same size and shape as an erythrocyte. Attached forms are difficult to see on fresh scrapes, but usually easy to see on histological preparations.

Table 1:
Classification of ectoparasitic protozoa.

FLAGELLATES (Possess flagella; may or may not contain chlorophyll)

    1. Flagellates - not containing chlorophyll

        Ichthyobo sp.   - Costiasis
        Cryptobia
        Hexamita   - Hole-in-the-Head disease

    2. Flagellates - at least one life cycle stage contains chlorophyll

        Amyloodinium sp. (Marine) $\Big\}$ - Velvet or Rust
        Oodinium Sp. (Freshwater)

CILIATES

    1. Holotrichous Ciliates - body uniformly covered in cilia

        Ichthyophthirius multifiliis $\Big\}$ - White Spot or Ich
        Cryptocaryon sp. (Marine)

        Tetrahymena corlissi $\Big\}$ - Tet Disease or Guppy killer
        Uronema sp. (marine)

        Chilodonella sp. $\Big\}$
        Brooklynella sp. (Marine)

    2. Peritrichous Ciliates - cilia present in only specialised groups

        Trichodinids
        Scyphidia complex

    3. Suctorian Ciliophora - these have suctorial tentacles instead of cilia

        Trichophyra

Treatment - General treatment as for all parasites. Formalin baths should kill the parasite.

Cryptobia

These organisms are mainly associated with cichlids and ciprinids, but may be seen on other fresh water and marine fish.

Characteristics - Very similar in appearance to costia but more elongated. They are found on gills and skin, and in the gastro-intestinal tract. They are thought to occur in the blood stream as trypanoplasms (see under blood parasites). The life cycle is direct.

Disease - Although some authorities consider these organisms to be commensals on the gills, they may cause damage. They are thought able to invade the body (see under Viscera and Musculature).

Diagnosis - Identification of the organism in gill, skin and/or gut scrapes.

Treatment - General treatment as for all parasites. Formalin baths should kill the external stages of these parasites.

Figure 1:
***Ichthyobodo* sp. (10μm in length). The figure shows attached form (highlighted with arrow) on primary lamellar tip of gill.**

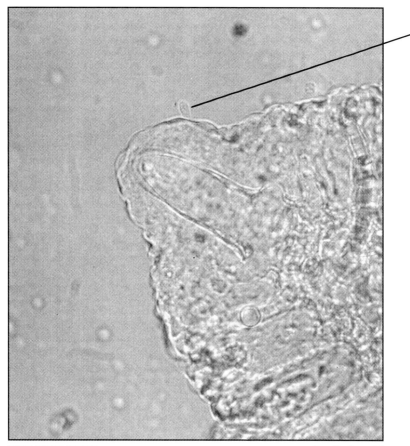

Photo: Edward Branson   Magnification x400

Hexamita

Thought to be the causative agent of **hole-in-the-head disease**. (See under Gastro-Intestinal Tract).

Amyloodinium sp. (Velvet Disease)

Also called **rust disease**, **gold dust disease**, **pillularis** and **coral fish disease**. The main organisms concerned are *Amyloodinium* sp. in salt water, and *Oodinium* sp. in fresh water. They are only found in warm waters and are usually a problem of tropical aquaria.

Characteristics - These organisms all contain chlorophyll at some stage of their life cycle. The parasitic stage is the trophont, 50-100μm in size, which can attach to the skin, gill and occasionally to the gut. This appears as a dark sac-like body, with granular cytoplasm, but with one end clear, this being the attachment area. Trophonts of some species contain chlorophyll. Eventually this detaches and forms a cyst, off the host, which divides to produce many dinospores, or 'swarmers'. These dinospores swim, by means of two flagella, to find a host; they are 12-15μm in size, and have chlorophyll and a red spot (the stigma) within the cytoplasm. Severe damage is caused at the site of attachment with inflammation, occasionally haemorrhage, and necrosis. They are not host specific and the life cycle is direct.

Disease - Skin and mainly gill damage are found with the typical signs of external parasitism. If present in sufficient numbers, they can appear as a gold or rust coloured velvety layer over the affected areas, (this colour being due to the chlorophyll), hence the disease names.

Diagnosis - Gross appearance and presence of parasites on skin and gill scrapings.

Treatment - General treatment as for all parasites. Chemical treatment is difficult, but copper sulphate is the commonest in use. Great care must be exercised when this is used in marine systems. U-V light can kill dinospores. Marine species are usually sensitive to fresh water (not brackish).

CILIATES

Ichthyophthirius multifiliis (White Spot)

Ichthyophthirius multifiliis causes a condition known as '**white spot**', '**ich**', or '**itch**'. This disease is extremely common, occurring in all freshwater fish species worldwide, although some species seem to be more resistant to its effects than others. A marine equivalent disease is caused by *Cryptocaryon* sp.

Characteristics - These organisms have a direct life cycle, but part of it is spent off the host. The tomite is the infective stage, ciliated, pear shaped, free swimming, 30-45μm in size and actively seeking a host; they die quite quickly if they are not successful (within 48hrs at 24 - 26°C). Once on the host, it penetrates the epidermis and develops into the trophont - the 'white spot'. The mature trophont is spherical, up to 1mm in diameter, uniformly ciliated all over its body, and has a characteristic horseshoe shaped nucleus. Within the skin it is active, consuming cellular material and causing irritation. Once mature, it leaves the fish, encysts and produces up to 2000 tomites. These tomites are released, and the whole cycle begins again. Life cycle length varies with temperature.

Disease - Typical signs of external parasitism with characteristic white spots on the skin and gills. The escape of the mature trophont causes epidermal damage which, if severe, may give rise to osmotic disturbance, haemorrhage and secondary infection. Infestations can build up very quickly in warm conditions.

Diagnosis - Appearance of white spots and the presence of tomites and/or trophonts in skin and/ or gill scrapes.

Treatment - General treatment as above for all parasites. The free swimming stages are the only parts of the life cycle susceptible to chemical treatment. The treatment usually used in fresh water is malachite green, alone or in combination with formalin. These chemicals will both destroy tomites, and have some effect on mature trophonts once outside the body. In sea water, copper based compounds may be used. Due to the inability of a single treatment to kill all life cycle stages, treatment must be repeated (usually 3 times) at intervals. The timing of these intervals is dependent on the length of the life cycle, which in turn depends on the water temperature (life cycle takes about 6 days at 27°C, about 15 days at 15°C). Early treatment is important due to the capacity of the organism to multiply so quickly.

As a general rule, 3 treatments should be given at:

>   5 day intervals at > 16°C
>   7 day intervals at 10-16°C
>   14 day intervals at < 10°C

Treatment of the water using ultra-violet filters will kill tomites. Quarantine is important to ensure that the disease is recognised before new fish are introduced into the system. Cysts may be attached to water plants, rocks, etc, so any new materials should also be quarantined. Any tomites emerging, will die after two or three days. Exposure to a low level of infection seems to produce some immunity.

Figure 2:
***Ichthyophythirius multifiliis.* The figure shows two large trophonts (approximately 400μm in diameter) and one small trophont (approximately 200μm in diameter).**

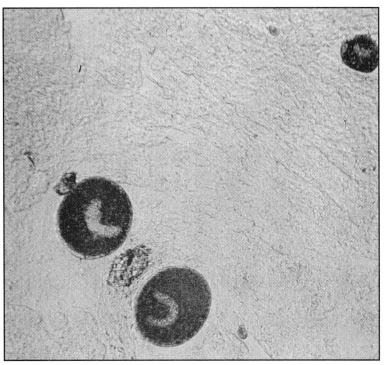

Photo: Edward Branson   Magnification x40

Tetrahymena

Tetrahymena corlissi is the cause of **Tet disease**, otherwise known as the **Guppy killer**, and can be another cause of **slime disease**. This is a warm water disease, and guppies and other live-bearers are most notably susceptible.

Characteristics - *T corlissi* is normally free living, but can parasitise fish. The organism is pear shaped, and similar in size and appearance to the infective tomites of Ich (approximately 60 μm in length). It has a direct life cycle and can reproduce on the host. A marine form of this disease can occur, caused by *Uronema* sp.

Disease - The parasites tend to swarm in particular areas on the fish, so white patches may be seen. Usually only stressed, or debilitated individuals are affected; females seem to be more susceptible than males, but severe disease may occur with no apparent predisposing cause. The parasite can invade most organ systems, leading to rapid mortality. Muscle swelling may be the only visible lesion. Deep ulcers may also occur, with invasion of the parasites into the musculature.

Diagnosis - Appearance of affected fish. Fresh scrapes will show large numbers of the organism. These may be distinguished from Ich by the lack of large trophonts in the scraping, and from *Chilodonella* sp. because they are not flattened.

Treatment - General treatment as for all parasites. Chemical treatment with formalin should kill them outside the host. There is no treatment for the organisms within the fish.

Chilodonella

These organisms are found worldwide and can affect all species of freshwater fish. They are particularly common on freshwater aquarium fish, are found on the skin and gills, and are another cause of **slime disease**. A marine equivalent, *Brooklynella* sp., occurs.

Characteristics - *Chilodonella* sp. are motile ciliates which are usually very active, typically flattened, heart shaped and approximately 30-70 μm in length. They have parallel rows of cilia along the body, an oral opening surrounded by cilia, and an obvious large oval nucleus. Movement is by a characteristic 'flipping' motion. They feed on plankton and cellular debris, and in so doing cause irritation. Any problem in the fish which increases the amount of food material available, such as debility, overcrowding or poor water quality, will lead to an increase in the parasite population. Large numbers, once present, cause irritation and more damage. The life cycle is direct and can occur entirely on the host.

Disease - Signs typical of external parasitism. Ragged fins may be seen.

Diagnosis - General clinical symptoms and identification of the organism in fresh skin or gill scrapes.

Treatment - General treatment as for all parasites. Chemical treatment with formalin baths.

Figure 3:
***Chilodonella* sp. Approximate size 50μm in diameter.**

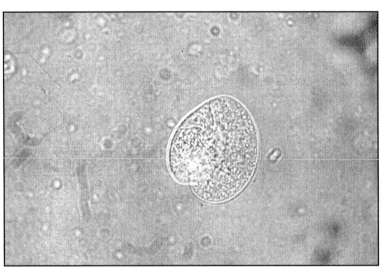

Photo: Edward Branson   Magnification x400

Trichodinids

Introduction - Three genera, *Trichodina* sp., *Trichodonella* sp., and *Tripartiella* sp., make up the trichodinid group. They are found worldwide, can affect all species of freshwater and marine fish, and can occur on the skin and gills. They are one of the causes of **slime disease**.

Characteristics - Trichodinids are saucer or bell shaped, approximately 40-100 μm in size. They contain a complicated arrangement of hook-like structures which give them a very characteristic appearance when seen in fresh preparations. The rim of the saucer is fringed with cilia which produce spinning motion. They move freely over the body surfaces attaching and detaching regularly. This process causes damage to host epidermal cells, and the resulting debris is consumed along with other debris present on the host or in the water. Even relatively small numbers can cause significant amounts of damage. They have a direct life cycle which can occur entirely on the host.

Disease - Signs typical of external parasitism. Fins may become ragged.

Diagnosis - General clinical symptoms and identification of the parasite on fresh skin or gill scrapes. Trichodinids are very characteristic.

Treatment - General treatment as for all parasites. Chemical treatment with formalin baths.

Figure 4:
Trichodinid. Approximate size 70μm in diameter.

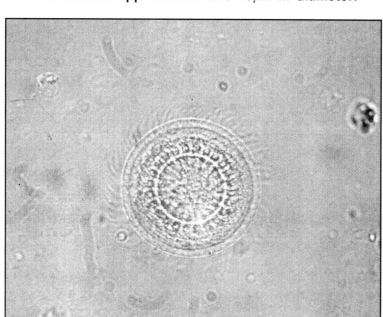

Photo: Edward Branson   Magnification x400

Scyphidia complex

Many species of scyphidians exist and are found worldwide. All species of freshwater and marine fish can be affected.

Characteristics - These organisms are flask shaped with a spiral of cilia at one end. The other end attaches to the skin or the gills of the host. Different species have different characteristics: *Scyphidia* sp. tend to be oblong, *Epistylis* sp. have long thin stalks, *Vorticella* sp. have long contractile stalks. The stalks of *Epistylis* sp can be branched so that many organisms can originate from one base stalk. They are approximately 50μm in diameter, the stalk length being variable with the species. The life cycle is direct, and can occur on the host. These organisms are commensals, and feed by filtering organic matter from the water. Problems usually occur only when there is high organic loading in the water, in which case large numbers can build up and cause skin irritation.

Disease - Signs typical of external parasitism. Heavy infestations with *Epistylis* sp. can give the gross appearance of a fungal infection. These organisms have been implicated in ulcer formation, but it is more likely that colonisation of an existing ulcer and consequent retardation of healing is a more common feature.

Diagnosis - General clinical symptoms and examination of fresh skin or gill scrapes.

Treatment - General treatment as for all parasites, with special emphasis on improving water quality. Chemical treatment with formalin can be used if necessary.

Figure 5:
Scyphidian. Approximate size 25μm in diameter.

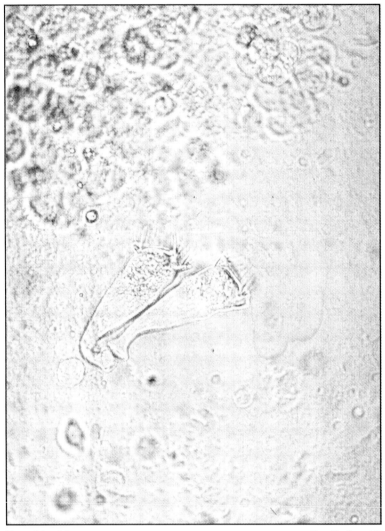

Photo: Edward Branson

Magnification x400

Trichophyra

These organisms occur worldwide and may be found on all species of freshwater and marine fish, although they are only seen with any regularity on the gills of fresh water fish.

Characteristics - *Trichophyra* sp. are rounded in shape, slightly granular in appearance, and have suctorial tentacles rather than cilia. These can be withdrawn and so may not be seen on microscopic examination. Their size is up to approximately 30 μm in diameter, and some may contain orange pigment granules. The life cycle is direct, and can occur entirely on the host, usually on the gills. They are commensals, and simply filter organic material from the water. As with scyphidians, they only usually become a problem with high organic loading in the water.

Disease - Pathological effect is doubtful, but if present on the gills in large numbers, may cause asphyxiation. Irritation may also occur, with consequent general signs of gill parasitism.

Diagnosis - General clinical symptoms and examination of fresh skin or gill scrapes. The suctorial tentacles will usually be withdrawn after the scrape is taken, but may be extended again after a while.

Treatment - As for scyphidians.

Figure 6:
Tricophyra sp. Approximate size 30μm in diameter.

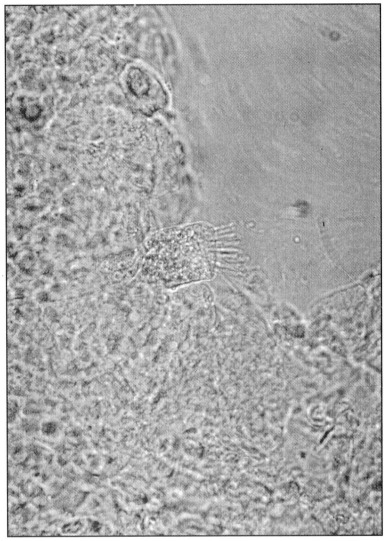

Photo: Edward Branson   Magnification x400

ENDOPARASITIC PROTOZOA

As with external protozoans, a small number of parasites in the gut may be considered normal, but with poor health of the host or adverse environmental conditions leading to stress and immunosuppression, explosive increases in numbers can occur with resulting disease.

General Signs

Symptoms will vary with the part of the body affected, but fish may show a general unthriftiness. When a specific organ is affected, specific symptoms related to that organ will probably occur. Intestinal parasitism may give rise to excessive mucus production resulting in translucent faeces. Swellings, or open lesions, may be seen if skin or muscle are affected. In the case of open lesions, secondary infection may occur, thus obscuring the primary aetiology.

Some infestations can be treated with chemicals, but mostly management is the only method of control. Quarantine, as for ectoparasites, is advisable for new introductions. However, many of the endoparasites are slower to develop than ectoparasites, and so may not become apparent within the normal quarantine period.

Disease Organisms

The main endoparasitic groups of Protozoa can be classified as follows:

Table 2:
Classification of endoparasitic protozoa

Parasites of the Gastro-Intestinal Tract

    1. Flagellates - not containing chlorophyll

        Hexamitids
        Coccidia

Parasites of the Viscera and Musculature

    1. Flagellates

        Cryptobia sp.- Malawi or Cichlid bloat

    2. Microspora

        Glugea sp.
        Pleistophora hyphessobryconis - Neon Tetra Disease

    3. Myxozoa
        Henneguya sp.
        Myxobolus sp.

Parasites of the Blood

        Trypanasomes
        Trypanoplasms

PARASITES OF THE GASTRO-INTESTINAL TRACT

Flagellates

Hexamitids

These organisms are found in the alimentary tract, and have been reported in a variety of species worldwide. Various genera occur, the best known being *Hexamita* sp., previously called *Octomitis* sp. Disease is usually only seen in fresh water species, but marine species can be affected.

Characteristics - *Hexamita* sp are pyriform to round in shape, approximately 5 x 10 μm long. They have three pairs of anterior and one pair of posterior flagella. Movement is rapid, usually in straight lines. Infection is probably by the oral route, and the organism establishes itself in the intestine or caeca, where it is free swimming. Haematogenous spread to other organs may occur. The life cycle occurs entirely on the host, but encysted forms may be released with the faeces which can probably infect other fish.

Disease - Large numbers of the parasite may cause unthriftiness and consequently increase mortality rate, but large numbers can be found in healthy fish with no apparent ill effects. It is likely that stress or underlying debility is necessary to precipitate disease. Conditions associated with these organisms include **Necrotic ulcerative gastritis** in Siamese fighting fish, with a related **granulomatous peritonitis**. Haematogenous spread to other organs may also occur. They have also been linked with **sudden death of young cichlids**, such as angel fish and gouramis, and, in association with *Capillaria* nematodes, with **severe enteritis** in angel fish.

Hole-in-the-head disease, especially seen in cichlids such as oscars and discus fish, has also been associated with these organisms, but a causal relationship has never been proven and nutritional factors are probably involved. This condition is characterised by severe multi-focal ulcerative dermatitis, especially on the head where lesions may extend deeply into the cranium. The most likely access of these parasites to these areas is by haematogenous spread from the gut. Carp may also suffer from an **ulcerative enteritis** of the posterior intestine due to similar organisms.

Diagnosis - General clinical symptoms along with observation of the organism in fresh scrapings taken from the caeca or intestine. In the case of 'hole-in-the-head disease', the organism can be seen in fresh scrapings of the skin lesions. Translucent faeces may occur due to excess mucus production. They are almost impossible to see unless moving, so fresh preparations are very important.

Treatment - The underlying health of the fish should be improved. Chemical treatment with, for example, dimetranidazole or furazolidone should kill the organisms.

Coccidia

Coccidia are found worldwide in many species of fish. In common with most other parasites, disease usually only occurs when the fish is subjected to stress. Very few occurrences of coccidiosis have been reported, these mainly in carp.

Characteristics - Various species of coccidia may be involved, mainly from the genus *Eimeria*. Most occur in the intestinal or caecal epithelium, but a few may be found in other organs. Infection usually begins with ingestion of the oocyte, which is the only stage of the life cycle to occur outside the host. The resulting sporozoites invade gut epithelial cells and begin reproduction, eventually producing oocytes which continue the cycle.

Disease - Signs include emaciation, lethargy and general poor health. Within the gut infestations are either diffuse (which may result in enteritis), or nodular (*E subepithelialis*, for example, produces white nodules in the intestine of carp). Faeces may be fluid and light in colour.

Diagnosis - Clinical signs along with the identification of the oocysts in faeces or caecal scrapes at x400 magnification. In fish with clinical coccidiosis, many oocysts will be present in faeces, but in non-clinical cases oocyst concentration may be necessary. Histological examination of gut sections will show the various stages of reproduction.

Treatment - General treatment as for all parasites. No chemical treatment has been evaluated, but coccidiostats used for terrestrial animals may be of use. The presence of a fine mesh screen over the bottom of the tank in order to stop fish picking up oocytes may help to prevent spread.

PARASITES OF THE VISCERA AND MUSCULATURE

Flagellates

Cryptobia (See Ectoparasite section).

Disease - In some cases these organisms may be capable of invading the stomach of cichlids, giving rise to granulomata in the submucosa and elsewhere. The spread is probably haematogenous. In combination with other pathogens, they may be associated with **Malawi or cichlid bloat**. One species has been found to concentrate in the gills, especially of carp, causing severe gill damage.

Diagnosis - Clinical appearance and identification of the parasite where possible.

Treatment - There is no treatment for the internal form.

Microspora

Many species of these organisms occur worldwide in a wide variety of fish. Some typical infections are: *Glugea* sp. in sticklebacks and *Pleistophora* sp. in neon tetras and golden shiners. *P hyphessobryconis* is the cause of **Neon Tetra disease**.

Characteristics - The microsporidia are intracellular parasites spores of which infect the host, probably by the oral route. A target cell is infected and develops into a trophozoite which, in time, produces large numbers of spores. The spores, which are Gram positive, consist of a small body approximately 2 x 3 µm, containing a polar capsule which stains strongly with Giemsa.

Disease - These organisms cause chronic conditions characterised by the slow growth of trophozoites which form boil-like masses within the tissues. These masses may cause deformities and interfere with movement, but otherwise do not usually have a significant effect on the host unless some vital organ is involved. Usually only individual fish are affected. Sub-dermal trophozoites can appear as grey swellings, and may rupture leaving open wounds. Terminal cases may become emaciated and lethargic, and may show abnormal colouration. Infections in gonads may reduce spawning success. *P hyphessobryconis* in **Neon Tetra disease** usually shows up as a loss of colour with milky white areas under the skin, usually along the dorsum, due to the trophozoites in the dorsal musculature.

Diagnosis - Appearance of trophozoites and the identification of spores - either in unstained or stained fresh preparations. Histological examination will also demonstrate spores.

Treatment - There is no therapy for this condition. Affected fish should be removed in an attempt to reduce spread to other fish. Spores are not usually shed until infected fish die, but this can occur earlier if trophozoites rupture to the outside through the skin or gut. Disinfection of the tank may be of use. The presence of a fine mesh screen over the bottom of the tank in order to stop fish picking up spores may help to prevent spread. All incoming fish should be quarantined, but due to the chronic nature of the condition, evidence of infection will probably not appear within the normal quarantine period.

Myxozoa

Many genera of Myxosporidia have been known to affect fish, and they are found worldwide, in fresh and salt water. They are usually extracellular parasites and occur in two forms:

i. Coelozoic (found in the swimbladder, urinary or gall bladders), and

ii. Histozoic (found in intercellular spaces of tissues).

Most of the organisms found in fish do not cause problems, but some are pathogenic.

Characteristics - As with microsporidia, the infective unit is the spore, but these are larger (in the region of 7 µm in diam.). The exact size, shape and structure of the spore (including the number and shape of strongly Giemsa staining polar capsules) is the primary means of identification of the myxosporidian. Infection is probably via the oral route. The spore is then thought to release a motile form into the blood stream which enters the target tissue and forms a trophozoite. Within this trophozoite, replication takes place resulting in many spores, or pre-spore stages, which are eventually released.

Disease - *Henneguya* sp. can infect various fish, amongst them carp and stickleback, and *Myxobolus* sp. are not uncommon in carp. Characteristically there are microscopic or larger opaque masses in various organs of the body, the site depending on the species of parasite, but this can include skin and gills. There may be no effect on the host, depending on the organ affected, but debility may occur. Rupture of sub-cutaneous trophozoites can result in open wounds.

A Sphaerospora-like myxosporean has been associated with **swim bladder inflammation** in carp, a pre-spore stage of this parasite being found in the swim bladder of affected fish. The parasites then move to the kidney via the blood. Signs include severe haemorrhage and necrosis of the epithelial lining of the swim bladder with, usually, some kidney swelling and peritonitis.

Severe kidney pathology in goldfish and other cyprinids has been found with infections of *Mitraspora cyprini*.

Diagnosis - Clinical appearance and the identification of typical spores in the lesions. Blood forms may be found in the bloodstream.

Treatment - There is no known therapy for myxosporidian infections. Control may be effected by the same techniques as recommended for microsporidia.

PARASITES OF THE BLOOD

Trypanosomes

These are not uncommon in both fresh and salt water. They may not be host specific, and few appear to be pathogenic.

Characteristics - Typical trypanosome morphology, 30-40 µm long. They are transmitted by a leech vector within which massive reproduction occurs. Different morphological forms exist within the fish and leech.

Disease - Anaemia with damage to the haemopoietic organs has been described in the goldfish. Death may follow.

Diagnosis - Identification of the organism within the bloodstream.

Treatment - No treatment known.

Trypanoplasms

These may be present in healthy fish, and only apparently cause disease under conditions of stress. They probably need a leech vector, and some may need a leech to complete their life cycle. They are generally thought to be the blood forms of *Cryptobia*.

Characteristics - Similar in appearance to Trypanosomes but with two flagella.

Disease - Vascular and inflammatory lesions have been reported in goldfish. Fish may be lethargic and swim abnormally. Superficial ulceration and blood loss may occur due to the leech vector.

Diagnosis - Identification of the organism within the blood stream.

Treatment - No treatment known.

CHAPTER NINE

METAZOAL PARASITES

Edward J Branson
Peter J Southgate

GENERAL CONSIDERATIONS

Some metazoans exist on fish as parasites but, in contrast to protozoans, are unlikely to be found as commensals. Although multicellular and consequently much larger than the protozoa, in some cases, such as gill flukes, low numbers on a fish can still be considered normal. Only when numbers become excessive, usually due to some imbalance in the fish, do problems occur. In other cases, such as anchor worms, even small numbers can cause severe problems. Generally, but not invariably, diseases due to metazoan parasites tend to be chronic.

There are no symptoms of disease that are really common to all the metazoans, although increased levels of mucus and 'flashing' are not uncommon. Symptoms are discussed in relation to each organism.

The same general rules apply to diseases caused by metazoans with respect to prevention and treatment, as to those caused by protozoa (Chapter 8). Quarantine of new fish should be carried out for a minimum of 4 weeks, and treatment of disease should be aimed at improving the underlying environmental conditions and health of the fish, and reduction of parasite numbers.

Most of the significant metazoan parasites of fish are considered below. Those described have direct life cycles except where indicated. In these cases, examples of simplified typical group life cycles are given at the beginning of each taxonomic section, and this life cycle applies to each member of that group unless otherwise indicated.

Non-Parasitic Metazoa

Other metazoans which may appear in aquaria, but which are not parasitic, are the Planarians, a group of free living Platyhelminthes, and *Hydra* sp. which belong to the Coelenterate group.

The Planarians may be up to 1cm in length and from white to red in colour. These organisms feed on detritus, but may consume eggs. Blooms can occur in poor conditions. Control can usually be maintained by good hygiene.

Hydra sp. can be up to 2cm in length, are similar in appearance to sea anemones, and can retract in the same way. They may colonise large areas of the tank surfaces and can kill, and consume, fish fry. A one week treatment with 0.5% salt solution should control the organism. Good hygiene should prevent reappearance.

ECTOPARASITIC METAZOA

The common groups of ectoparasitic metazoa are listed below:

Platyhelminthes
 	
        Monogenean trematodes (Flukes)
                Dactylogyrus sp. - Gill Fluke
                Gyrodactylus sp. - Skin Fluke

Mollusca   Glochidia

Crustacea (Class within Arthropoda)
 	
        Copepoda
                Lernaea sp. -   Anchor Worms
                Ergasilus sp. -   Gill Maggots
 	
        Branchiura
                Argulus sp. -   Fish Lice

Annelida   *Piscicola* sp. -   Leeches

MONOGENEAN TREMATODES

Monogeneans have a worldwide distribution and may be found on most freshwater and marine species, although they are probably more common in fresh water. Most are host specific although some cross infection may occur. They can be a cause of **slime disease**, and include the **skin and gill flukes**.

Characteristics - These parasites are found on the skin or gill, and browse on the body surface. They attach by means of posterior hooks, which cause significant tissue damage, and an anterior sucker. They are either oviparous or viviparous, and typical of these groups are *Dactylogyrus* sp. and *Gyrodactylus* sp. respectively. Sizes range from 0.1 to 2mm in length. Infection is by direct contact or, in the case of the oviparous group, by free swimming larvae arising from the eggs.

Dactylogyrus sp. are often found on the gills (although not exclusively) and are known as **gill fluke**. Eggs are produced which fall from the host, hatch, and then infect a new host. Orange/brown vitelline glands and eye spots are usually visible within the body.

Gyrodactylus sp. are most commonly found on the skin, and are known as **skin fluke**. These have no eye spots. Within the body cavity juveniles can be seen, recognisable by the presence of posterior hooks, and often these juveniles themselves contain further juveniles. The young are released onto the host, so no stage of the life cycle need leave the host. Due to this process, parasite numbers can build up very quickly under the right circumstances. Generation times are temperature dependent, and at low temperatures (1-2°C) can be as long as 6 months.

Other organisms belonging to this group may be seen, but generally their characteristics are similar to those described above.

Figure 1:
Gyrodactylus sp. containing juvenile. Approximate size 600µm in length.

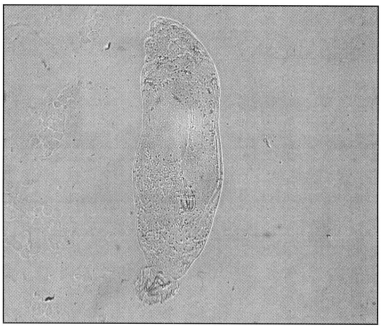

Photo: Edward Branson   Magnification: X 100

Disease - Disease signs will depend on the area of body affected. Generally there will be increased mucus production, with consequent greyness of affected areas. Noticeable grey areas, especially around the fins, are characteristic. If the gills are affected, there will be evidence of respiratory distress. 'Flashing' and rubbing is common in the early stages, with lethargy, listlessness, anorexia, and, possibly, mucus depletion later. Damage caused by the parasites may cause petechiation, especially in the gills, and osmoregulatory imbalance. These changes predispose to secondary bacterial or fungal infection.

Diagnosis - Clinical symptoms and the presence of the organisms on fresh gill or skin scrapes. Distinction between the two types is important for the purposes of treatment.

Treatment - Correct the underlying husbandry problems. If oviparous species are involved, cleaning and sterilisation of tanks may be useful. Chemical treatments should bring the problem under control, and use of formalin may be adequate. Marine species respond well to reversed salinity. Organophosphates or other chemicals have been used where formalin has failed. One treatment may be enough to control viviparous species, but with oviparous species there is likely to be reinfection, so re-treatment will probably be necessary.

Figure 2:
Dactylogyrus sp. on gill squash.

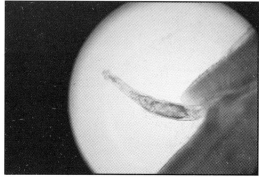

Photo: Ray Butcher   Magnification: X 20

MOLLUSCA

This group is not usually significant, but larval stages (glochidia) of fresh water mussels are parasitic, and could be a problem in fish held in ponds fed from streams with mussel beds.

Characteristics - The glochidia may attach to gills, fins and skin and become encysted. Problems can occur with heavy infestations interfering with respiration, but the main effect is usually seen when the larvae leave the host. Significant damage can be caused as this occurs, and osmotic problems and secondary infections can follow.

Disease - Respiratory distress.

Diagnosis - Presence of white nodular swellings on the gill filaments.

Treatment - None known.

COPEPODA (A group within the Class Crustacea)

The main genus of interest in this group is *Lernaea*, the **anchor worms**. *L cyprinacea* is a parasite of carp, but it is not host specific. It occurs in fresh water in Europe, North America and Asia. It is more important in warm water, and is unable to complete it's life cycle below 15°C. Other species occur in other environments, including some in salt water, but do not usually cause problems. Another genus which may occasionally be seen is *Ergasilus* sp., the **gill maggots** of fresh and salt, usually warm, water.

Characteristics - The female anchor worm is fertilised on the host's body to which it then attaches and undergoes a metamorphosis. The result of this is that the head is thrust through the host's body wall and forms a cephalic process, leaving the posterior part of the body outside the host's body. This cephalic process has almost the appearance of a 'root system' within the body of the host, and forms an anchor for the parasite, hence the common name. Egg sacs are formed on the posterior part of the body and trail in the water, releasing eggs which hatch into nauplii. Their development occurs first off, and then on, the body of the potential host until they are about 1mm in length, when mating takes place. The male dies, and the female then begins the anchoring process. These parasites can be up to 22mm long when fully grown. Transmission is via water supply or by introduction of infected fish. Attachment of early stages to amphibians or birds may play a part.
Ergasilids are much smaller, up to 3mm long when fully grown. They attach themselves to gills by means of a pair of claspers which cause gill damage, and have pairs of characteristic trailing egg sacs.

Disease - Even small numbers of anchor worms will cause serious damage to the host, and can cause rapid death if vital organs are affected. Evidence of parasitic infestation such as 'flashing' may indicate an early problem, but other concurrent diseases should be ruled out. With heavy infestations fish may show lethargy, listlessness, unthriftiness, etc, and there may be secondary infection with bacteria or fungi. Sites of parasitic attachment are usually inflamed, sometimes producing a tumour-like mass. After the parasite has fallen away, these wounds are slow to heal.

Ergasilids will cause severe gill damage due to the claspers, with consequent evidence of gill disease.

Diagnosis - Adult anchor worms are very obvious, protruding from the skin of the host, and ergasilids can easily be seen in the gill cavities. Both have characteristic trailing paired egg sacs, although quite small in the latter case.

Treatment - Control of anchor worm is probably best achieved by removal of larval stages in the water by use of organophosphates and the mechanical removal of egg laying adults, which are not sensitive to organophosphates. Provided all egg laying adults are removed, one, or possibly two, organophosphate treatments should be adequate. Ulcers resulting from infection should be suitably treated. All stages of the anchor worm life cycle are sensitive to drying, including eggs, and will die after 24hrs. Therefore draining and drying of infected systems will eliminate the parasite, as long as egg producing females are removed. Fish recovering from infestation by these parasites may have some immunity to reinfection.

Pond treatment with organophosphates is also the method of treatment for ergasilids, both adults and juveniles being sensitive in this case.

BRANCHIURA (A group within the Class Crustacea)

The most important member of this group is the genus *Argulus*. Otherwise known as **fish lice**, these parasites are found worldwide in all types of water. In Europe they are primarily associated with fresh water problems, and are not host specific. They usually hibernate on the body of the host below 8°C, and egg production ceases below about 16°C.

Characteristics - This parasite is dorso-ventrally flattened with obvious eye-spots, oval in shape, and 5 to 10mm in length. It has hooks and suckers for attachment, and feeding is via a stylet, all of which cause damage to the host. They are almost transparent and can move around on the fishes body very quickly. Male and female live on the host until the female is ready to lay eggs, at which time she drops off and deposits eggs on aquatic plants. After this she returns to a host. Three to four days after hatching the second copepodid stage finds a host, and continues to metamorphose until adulthood. The entire life cycle takes 40 to 100 days depending on temperature. Transmission is via water supply or by introduction of infected fish. Attachment of early stages to amphibians or birds may play a part.

Disease - Obvious evidence of irritation occurs, such as 'flashing' and rubbing. Heavily infested fish may be listless, lethargic and unthrifty. Sites of parasitic feeding may become abraded, are often haemorrhagic, and may suffer from secondary infection. There may be excessive mucus production. These parasites are thought to transmit viruses, such as Spring Viraemia of carp.

Diagnosis - Adult *Argulus* are easily seen on the surface of the fish.

Treatment - All stages of the life cycle are sensitive to drying, including eggs, and will die after 24hrs. Draining and drying of systems, therefore, will eliminate the parasite. Adult *Argulus* are very salt tolerant, but juveniles will be killed by concentrations of 2%. Adults and juveniles may be killed by use of organophosphates. Removal of sites for egg laying will reduce numbers of parasites hatching. Alternatively, special sites for egg-laying, such as branches, can be introduced, these being removed every day and allowed to dry out. Increasing water flow rates may reduce the level of infective stages.

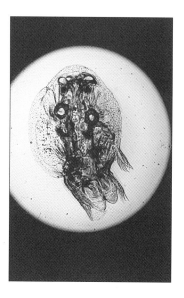

Figure 3:
***Argulus* sp.**
Magnification X 20

Photo: Ray Butcher

ANNELIDA

Leeches

Leeches are found worldwide in fresh and salt water.

Characteristics - Although many do not affect fish, some feed directly on fish blood. Reproduction occurs off the host, eggs being attached to any surface in the water.

Disease - During feeding damage occurs to skin and underlying tissues, with a consequent risk of osmotic regulatory problems and secondary infection. This damage is particularly important in small or debilitated fish. Leeches are known to act as intermediate hosts for certain blood parasites, such as trypanoplasms and trypanosomes, and may transmit the causative virus of Spring Viraemia of carp.

Diagnosis - Areas of skin haemorrhage on the fish and the presence of large numbers of leeches in the system.

Treatment - Treatment of the system with organophosphates should control the problem although eggs will not be eliminated by this method. Draining and drying the system should eliminate adults and eggs.

Fig 4 (a): Fish leech (*Piscicola* sp.)

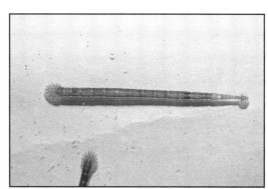

Photo: Ray Butcher

Fig 4 (b) Fish leech showing sucker

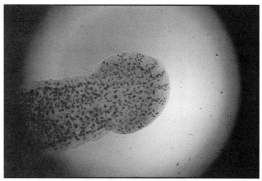

Photo: Ray Butcher   Magnification: X 20

ENDOPARASITIC METAZOA

The main groups of endoparasitic Metazoa, with some examples, are listed below:

Table 1:
Classification of endoparasitic metazoa.

Parasites of the Viscera and Musculature

    Platyhelminthes

        Digenean Trematodes (Flukes)
            Neascus sp. -   Black spot
            Diplostomum sp. - Eye fluke
            Clinostomum sp. - Yellow and white grubs

        Cestoda (Tapeworms)
            Ligula sp.
            Triaenophorus sp.
            Diphyllobothrium sp.

    Nematoda

            Philometra sp. -   Blood worms
            Eustrongyloides sp.

Parasites of the Gastro-Intestinal Tract

    Platyhelminthes

        Digenean Trematodes -   little importance

        Cestoda (Tapeworms)
            Bothriocephalus sp. - The Asian tapeworm

        Nematoda

            Capillaria sp.
            Camellanus sp.

        Acanthocephala (Thorny-headed worms)

            Pomphorhynchus sp.

Parasites of the Blood

    Platyhelminthes

        Digenean Trematodes
            Sanguinicola inermis

ENDOPARASITES OF THE VISCERA AND MUSCULATURE

Digenean trematodes

A generalised simplified life cycle of the group is shown below:

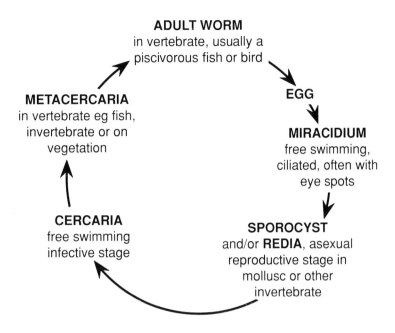

These organisms have complex life cycles, and fish may be involved as primary or intermediate hosts, depending on parasite species. They are found in fresh and salt water, and in all environmental conditions. Adult and metacercarial stages can occur in fishes, but the metacercarial stage is usually the most significant pathogen. These include **white** and **yellow grubs** seen throughout the body, **black spot** in the skin, and **eye fluke**. The most common to occur in fishes usually have a piscivorous bird as the final host. Where the adult stage occurs this is normally seen in the gut but can occur elsewhere eg. the blood – see later.

Figure 5:
***Diplostomum* sp. Approximately 440μm in length.**

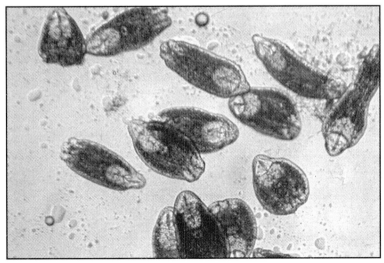

Photo: Edward Branson   Magnification: X 40

Characteristics - Most digeneans have a typical trematode life cycle and many involve fish in their life cycles, but only those of most interest are considered below. Once metacercaria are encysted within the fish, they are not usually a problem, although in the case of **eye fluke** permanent blindness may occur.

Disease - Invasion of fish by very large numbers of cercariae can cause osmotic disruption and death, especially in small fish. Symptoms will depend upon the species of parasite involved, and the site of the host affected, but in cases where an abnormal host is involved, there may be a massive inflammatory response.

Typical organisms found are:

Neascus sp. The cause of **black spot**, especially seen incyprinids. Metacercariae encyst in the skin and become melanised. Cysts can be up to 0.5mm or more in diameter.

Diplostomum sp. and others. The **eye flukes**, which can cause cataract and blindness because the eye is the target organ.

Clinostomum sp. The yellow or white grubs, notable for their size, 0.5cm or more in diameter. If these are near the surface of the body ulceration can occur.

Diagnosis - Diagnosis of a digenean infection is by recognition of the parasite. Usually there is little problem caused by a few digeneans within their natural host, but where problems do occur, identification of the species or group of parasite involved is necessary for successful control. Dissection of cysts , if their size allows, will usually demonstrate that metacercariae are present, but the actual identification of the species is extremely complex. Adult stages can sometimes be identified from taxonomic keys.

Treatment - In aquaria there is little chance of a life cycle being completed so once infection has been introduced it should not spread. Likely intermediate hosts should be avoided. There is no known effective chemical treatment for metacercariae in fish. If an infection is identified in a pond the best method of control is to break the life cycle of the parasite. Adult digeneans may be removed by use of therapeutic agents.

Figure 6:
Metacercaria within the gill of a Platy (*Xiphophorus maculatus*).

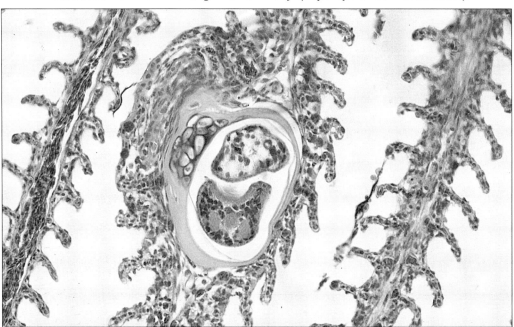

Photo: Ray Butcher   Magnification: X 200

76

CESTODA

A generalised, simplified life cycle of the group is shown below:

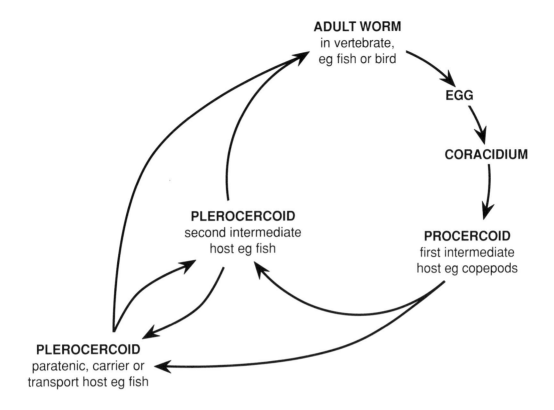

Cestodes, or tapeworms, occur in fish worldwide and in all types of environment. Many are host specific. Fish can be the final, intermediate or transport host, depending on species. Adult cestodes in fish are usually found in the gut, whereas intermediate stages may occur in any tissue or cavity. Usually these organisms cause very little harm to the host, except if present in large numbers.

Characteristics - The plerocercoid is the stage commonly found in the viscera, musculature, or even gut, of fishes. This stage is recognisable by the presence of an adult scolex. Sites of encystment within intermediate hosts depends on the species involved.

Disease - Large numbers of adult or intermediate cestodes within a fish may cause unthriftiness, with an increased susceptibility to other disease. If individual organs are affected there may be disease signs related to this organ. Generally, however, even large numbers of these parasites may not cause problems. Many occur in fish, some of interest are:

Ligula sp. Seen especially in cyprinids. The plerocercoid is found free within the abdominal cavity, and can be up to 20cm long and present in very large numbers. They can cause severe organ atrophy due to their bulk, and localised peritonitis. Affected fish may become lethargic, and sexual maturity may be inhibited.

Triaenophorus sp. The plerocercoid is found encysted in the liver of many species. The migratory phase can cause much damage.

Diphyllobothrium sp. The plerocercoid is usually found in the abdominal cavity, sometimes encysted, sometimes not. Other than some adhesions, little damage is caused once there. Some species may encyst in the muscle. Most damage is caused during the migratory phase before encapsulation takes place.

Diagnosis - Presence and identification of the causative organism. However due to the fact that large numbers of these organisms may not cause problems, the presence of any intercurrent disease should be determined. Intermediate stages which have been present within fish for long periods may appear as chronic granulomata, often with no parasitic tissue remaining.

Treatment - There is no known treatment for the intermediate stages of these parasites.

NEMATODA

A generalised, simplified life cycle for the group is shown below:

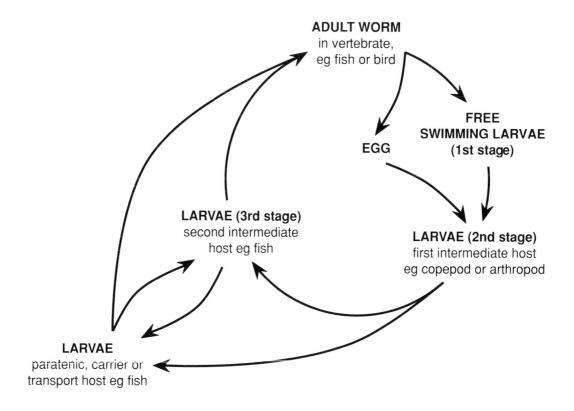

These organisms have a worldwide distribution, and are found in all environments. Many species of nematode can be carried by fish, either as the larval stage and/or the adult, but resultant disease is rare.

Characteristics - Nematodes found in fish are typical of the class. They are usually visible to the naked eye and fusiform in shape, ranging in size up to 2cms in length. They are usually host specific. Adult female nematodes release eggs into the water, either from the gut or through the skin. Fish may be final or intermediate hosts.

Disease - When nematode burdens become too large, evidence may include anaemia, emaciation, and unthriftiness, and fish may become susceptible to other diseases. Raised areas under the skin, or swellings in the musculature or other organs may be caused by cysts containing coiled larvae. Some larvae, especially if present within unnatural hosts, may wander and cause extensive tissue reaction, with resulting effects depending upon the organs damaged. Organisms of interest are:

Eustrongyloides sp. Larval stages are seen in fish. These are quite large, 8cm or more in length, red in colour so are easily seen, and found coiled up in fibrous capsules. The adult worm is found in piscivorous birds. They occur mainly in warmer waters and are relatively harmless.

Philometra sp. These nematodes, often called **blood worms**, are thin and red, up to 16cm long, and the adult females are found in the skin, fins, or lying free in the body cavity. They produce live larvae directly into the water by migrating to the superficial tissues and protruding the posterior part of their body through the skin; this then ruptures releasing larvae. The result of this is a superficial ulcer.

Diagnosis - Presence of the parasite. It is important to ensure that no intercurrent disease is present before a problem is attributed to nematode infestation. Old encysted nematode larvae may be seen by histological examination as calcified granulomata.

Treatment - Use of chemotherapeutics may kill adult worms, but no known treatment is available for larval stages. Removal of affected fish and cleaning and sterilisation of the system may help to reduce incidence by breaking the life cycle.

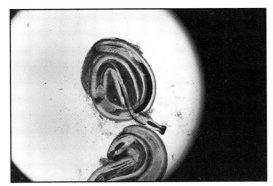

Photo: Ray Butcher   Magnification: X 20

Figure 7:
Encysted nematode larvae
from the peritoneal cavity
of a Platy (*Xiphophorus maculatus*).

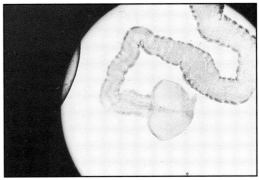

Photo: Ray Butcher   Magnification: X 20

Figure 8:
***Bothriocephalus* sp.**
from the small intestine of a koi.

ENDOPARASITES OF THE GASTRO-INTESTINAL TRACT

DIGENEAN TREMATODES

(See Viscera and Musculature section).

Disease - Adult digenean trematodes are not unusual findings in the gut of pond and aquarium fish, but none are thought to be pathogenic.

CESTODA

(See Viscera and Musculature section).

Disease - *Bothriocephalus* sp.(known as the **Asian tapeworm**). This can be up to 20cm in length, and is found as the adult form in the gut of carp. Infected fish have a swollen abdomen and may become sluggish and emaciated. Losses can occur due to the worm causing total blockage of the gut.

Diagnosis - Presence and identification of the parasite.

Treatment - Adult cestodes may respond to treatment with anthelmintics. Any treatment should include breaking the life cycle of the parasite, but this is unlikely to be relevant in an aquarium.

NEMATODA

(See Viscera and Musculature section)

Disease - *Capillaria* sp. These are generally thought of as pathogens of aquarium fish, causing gut ulceration and emaciation. Eggs are produced which are released directly into the environment. One species is found in the gut of Angel fish and cichlids. Affected fish cease to feed, often lie on their side, and may die. Faeces may appear translucent due to excessive mucus production. Another species particularly affects, and may kill, young armoured catfish if heavily infested.

Camellanus sp. These are common parasites of many live bearing tropical fish. They are thin red worms which may be seen protruding from the, possibly swollen, vent. They may be up to 1cm in length. Larvae may be carried in the tissues of, for example, *Daphnia* sp. Some species produce live larvae which do not need intermediate hosts, so heavy infestations can build up quite quickly. Damage to the intestine can occur with consequent ulceration.

Diagnosis - Presence and identification of the parasite. Gut scrapes may be necessary to see some species. Faecal smears may show the presence of *Capillaria* sp. eggs.

Treatment - Use of anthelmintics should remove adult worms.

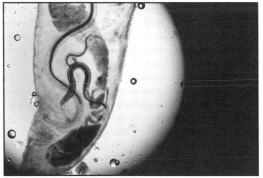

Photo: Ray Butcher   Magnification: X 20

Figure 9:
***Camellanus* sp. within the small intestine of a Platy (*Xiphophorus maculatus*).**

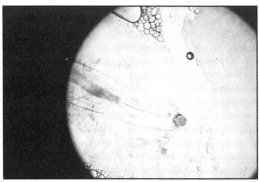

Photo: Ray Butcher   Magnification: X 80

Figure 10:
***Camellanus* sp. as in Figure 9, enlarged to show the head.**

ACANTHOCEPHALA

A generalised, simplified life cycle is shown below:

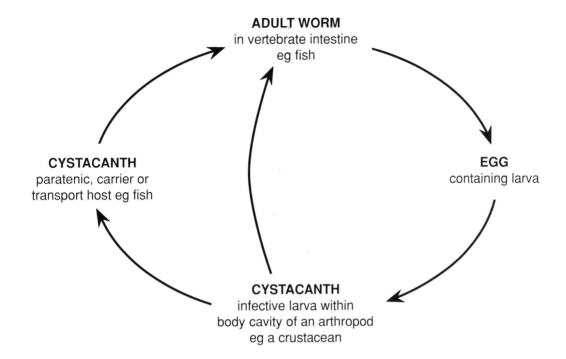

ADULT WORM
in vertebrate intestine
eg fish

EGG
containing larva

CYSTACANTH
infective larva within
body cavity of an arthropod
eg a crustacean

CYSTACANTH
paratenic, carrier or
transport host eg fish

These are the **thorny-headed worms** and are found worldwide. *Pomphorhynchus* sp. is a typical genus.

Characteristics - They are found in the digestive tract of vertebrates. Fish can be primary or reservoir hosts. The parasites are cylindrical in shape with a proboscis carrying a number of hooks which are used for attachment to the lining of the gut. The number and position of these hooks determines species. Those found in fishes may be up to 2 cm in length. Few are considered pathogenic.

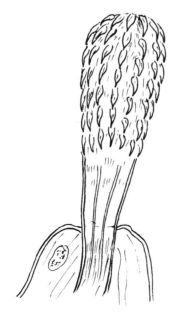

**Figure 11:
Proboscis of
Acanthocephala sp.**

Disease - These worms attach to the epithelium of the alimentary tract by means of the spiny head. This attachment causes damage to the gut lining which can result in ulceration, necrosis and possible perforation and peritonitis. Usually only the presence of large numbers of worms is pathogenic, but the presence of such large numbers may indicate some underlying problem in the host.

Diagnosis - Presence of the worm.

Treatment - Piperazine citrate may remove these parasites.

ENDOPARASITES OF THE BLOOD

DIGENEAN TREMATODES

(See Viscera and Musculature section)

Characteristics - *Sanguinicola inermis* is a potentially serious problem in carp. They enter the host as cercariae which do not form metacercariae, but continue to migrate around the body, usually remaining within the skin blood vessels. Near maturity, they migrate to the heart and then to the gill vessels where they lay eggs. The eggs are trapped in these vessels where they remain until hatching, when the miracidia burst out, thus causing serious gill damage. A mollusc is necessary for the completion of the life cycle. Some adults stay in the skin to lay eggs, so haemorrhages may be seen there, and some eggs are transported by the blood to other organs, especially the kidney, where the miracidia eventually result in granulomata formation.

Disease - Serious gill disease can occur, and secondary infections may be seen in the damaged gills. Liver and kidney damage may cause debility.

Diagnosis - Adult worms can be seen in the gills and heart, but they are easy to miss. Gills are usually swollen, with anaemic lamellae due to the blocked blood vessels. Eggs may be seen histologically in the gills, and also within granulomata in the kidneys.

Treatment - The anthelmintic drug praziquantel has been used to kill the adult worms, but the life cycle must also be interrupted. Supportive treatment should be given to fish affected by the egg release.

CHAPTER TEN

FUNGAL DISEASES

Edward J Branson
Peter J Southgate

GENERAL CONSIDERATIONS

Fungi tend to derive their nutritional requirements from dead organic matter but some can utilize living organisms in certain circumstances. The relative ease with which this can be done depends on the type of fungus.

A wide variety of fungi have been associated with disease in fish, usually occurring sporadically, sometimes as epizootics, sometimes as incidental findings.

Morphologically they vary from single celled organisms to those with hyphae. Hyphae are usually branched and tend to form a tangled mass, the mycelium. Some hyphae have obvious cell walls (septate), whereas others have none (aseptate). Most produce spores, sometimes motile, these being the primary unit of transmission. Many spores are resistant to heat, drying and disinfectants.

Fungal infections can vary from superficial problems with little clinical effect, to fulminating systemic disease. Between these extremes can be a range of conditions with varying degrees of pathological effect.

Generally most disease of this type is secondary, precipitated by poor environmental conditions, malnutrition or other primary disease. However, once an infection is present within an aquarium or pond, the level of infective material may increase dramatically to the point where even apparently healthy fish succumb to disease.

Consequently any treatment of fungal disease, as with any other infectious disease, must include the removal of infected fish, dead or alive, as soon as the disease is recognised. This process along with an improvement in underlying husbandry should help to reduce the further incidence of the disease.

Although many fungi have been found associated with disease, most are uncommon. The commonest fungal diseases to occur in fish are given below.

SAPROLEGNIASIS

This disease is common in fish and their eggs, especially as a condition secondary to physical damage. It occurs world wide, primarily in fresh water, but also in brackish water. It is not seen in the marine environment.

Characteristics - Members of the two main genera involved, *Saprolegnia* sp and *Achyla* sp, have long, branched, aseptate hyphae, approximately 20μm in diameter. They reproduce asexually and produce spherical biflagellate zoospores within long slender zoosporangia, which are of slightly larger diameter than the hyphae. These zoospores may encyst and produce many secondary zoospores, so they have a massive capacity for reproduction. Zoospores attach to damaged areas on the fish, germinate, and then grow to cover the injured site. Once the infection is established, the production of proteolytic enzymes causes further damage so that the fungus can spread to more normal adjacent tissue. Zoospores may be introduced to a system on the feathers of birds, in animal faeces, and by the wind as well as in the water. The temperature range is from 0°C to 35°C.

Disease - This is not a primary disease, but is secondary to other problems such as **fin rot**, **ulcer disease**, **white spot**, or physical damage such as may occur during handling. The infection starts superficially, but deeper invasion may occur. Eventually tufts of cotton wool-like material appear (the mycelium). This then spreads, and can result in osmoregulatory problems and ultimately death, which will occur quite rapidly if gills are involved. Dead fish are an ideal breeding ground for the fungus, and their presence will enormously increase the number of infective spores in the water. Dead fish eggs are another good site for fungal growth, and the resulting mycelium can spread out and engulf neighbouring healthy eggs. Suffocation and further egg death then follows.

These fungi, although associated primarily with disease of the epidermis and dermis, have been recorded in the central nervous system and brain of some small tropical fish and, on occasion, in other internal organs.

Diagnosis - The appearance of tufts of grey/white cotton wool-like material is typical, although they may appear brown or black due to entrapment of suspended solids. Fresh preparations should be examined in order to distinguish it from other conditions with a similar appearance, such as *Epistylis* and myxobacterial infection. Such examination should show branched aseptate hyphae; zoosporangia may be seen.

Treatment - Correction of underlying husbandry problems is very important. The level of infective spores should be reduced by removal of infected material. Salt or malachite green dips have been used to treat the condition. Local treatment may be used where appropriate.

BRANCHIOMYCOSIS

A fungal disease of gill tissue, also known as **gill rot**. It is not found world wide, being confined to Europe, Japan, India and parts of the USA. Probably all freshwater species are susceptible, but especially cyprinids.

Characteristics - Two species of fungus can be involved, *Branchiomyces sanguinis* and *B demigrans*. Both produce branched, aseptate hyphae, approximately 8-30μm in diameter. Asexual, non-motile spores are the main reproductive unit, and arise from swollen areas of hyphae. Temperature

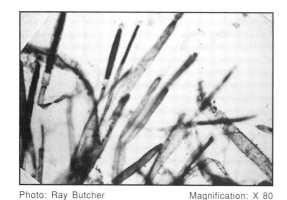

Photo: Ray Butcher   Magnification: X 80

Figure 1
Saprolegnia sp. showing hyphae

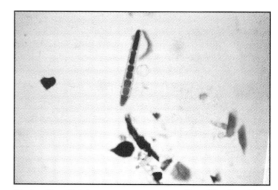

Photo: Ray Butcher   Magnification: X 80

Figure 2
Saprolegnia sp. showing zoosporangia

range is approximately 14-35°C, with optimum temperatures of 25-32°C at which epizootics can occur. Transmission is probably directly from the water to the gill. Spores attach to the gill surface, germinate, and hyphae penetrate the gill tissue. The gill blood supply is compromised, eventually causing necrosis. Necrotic tissue contains hyphae and spores which, when sloughed, releases spores into the water. Once shed, growth and reproduction can continue on the bottom of the pond or aquarium if conditions are right. Such conditions are those of high temperature, high levels of organic matter, low oxygen and low pH. Incubation period can be as little as 2 days. Spread is by the introduction of carriers, or infective material in the form of raw fish products. The spores may be carried on the feathers and legs of birds. Occasionally the fungus may occur in organs other than the gills, but this is not usually associated with problems.

Disease - Acute and sub-acute forms are characterised by lethargy and respiratory distress. Gills may appear bright red due to congestion, or white to brown depending on the stage of necrosis reached. Typically there is a 'marbled' appearance. In the sub-acute condition gills become ragged due to the sloughing of tissue, and gill arches may be present with no soft tissue left. Chronic infections can occur, and such carrier fish will probably show few signs.

Diagnosis - The appearance of the gill should be indicative of the condition - marbling, necrosis, and lack of soft tissue on gill arches. Phase microscopy may reveal the presence of hyphae and spores within the tissue.

Treatment - No treatment is known, but some authorities suggest that use of 2-phenoxyethanol may be beneficial. Once present in a system, control may be achieved by improving husbandry in order to provide good conditions for the fish, but adverse conditions for the organism. Levels of infective spores should also be reduced by good hygiene. Treatment of pond bottoms with quicklime or copper sulphate after draining may destroy the agent. Avoidance of the condition is best achieved by not using raw fish products, and not introducing infected fish.

ICHTHYOPHONIASIS

A systemic granulomatous disease found world wide in many fresh water and marine species. It has also been reported in some amphibians and copepods. Epizootics have occurred in wild species.

Characteristics - This condition is caused by *Ichthyophonus hoferi*, sometimes called *Ichthyosporidian* sp. It seems to be an obligate parasite with a complicated life cycle. The stage usually seen in the fish is the resting stage cyst, a spherical structure with a thick double wall, 10-250µm in diameter. These cysts are usually surrounded by a host connective tissue capsule forming nodules. Cyst contents appear amorphous, but in fact consist of many endospores. When the host dies, spores are released which can then infect a new host, usually by the oral route. Amoeboid bodies pass through the gut wall and are carried around the body by the blood. On coming to rest, they form another cyst. There may be local spread at this stage. Presence of the organism stimulates the host's response, usually a granulomatous reaction, which limits further spread and results in a well developed connective tissue capsule. Some infection may occur through wounds. As the initial spread is haematogenous, the organs with the greatest blood supply tend to be most affected. These are mainly heart, liver, kidney and spleen, but they can occur anywhere. Cysts will remain in the host for life, but if in the gut wall or skin, they may escape from the body earlier. The time from release to infectivity is thought to be in the region of one to six weeks. Viability within sediments can be for several years. Carriers are a potential source of infection, and infective forms may be carried into a system by birds. Copepods may also be involved.

Disease - A slight to moderate infection is unlikely to cause a problem, but scoliosis and lordosis have been reported, usually related to an effect on the nervous system rather than a local effect on the spine. Heavy infection can result in a 'sandpaper effect' in the skin, a condition where many lesions occur in the dermis giving the skin a rough texture. These lesions may be melanized, and may rupture leaving small ulcers. Extensive growth of the fungus can result in abscess formation due to local necrosis. Internally the organs may be swollen with grey/white/yellow nodular lesions. Mortality levels will depend on the level of infection and the organs affected.

Diagnosis - Diagnosis is based on the internal and external appearance, along with identification of the fungus. Other causes of granulomata should be considered as a differential diagnosis (infection by *Mycobacterium* sp. for example). Histopathology gives a definitive diagnosis, but microscopic examination of a fresh preparation from a lesion may show the presence of spherical bodies with double refractile walls, typical of the resting cysts.

Treatment - As for Branchiomycosis, but infected ponds may be very difficult to clear. Years of drying in sunshine may be necessary to ensure that all infective forms are destroyed.

DERMOCYSTIDIUM

There is some doubt over the classification of these organisms, but generally they are considered to be fungi. They occur in many species worldwide.

Characteristics - *Dermocystidium* sp can form cysts anywhere in the body but are commonly seen in the skin or gills. Cysts are usually smooth, yellowish/white, and can be up to 1cm or more in size. They are usually oval or round, but may be elongated. Cysts contain many thousand spores 3-6µm in diameter. Each spore has an eccentric nucleus, a large vacuole, and an inclusion body. The life cycle is unknown, but each organism may be specific to a small number of species.

Disease - Usually seen as yellow/white nodules in the skin or gills. Heavy infestations may be debilitating, especially if present in the gill when respiratory distress may occur. Low levels of infection probably cause no harm. *D. koi* forms cysts in the dermis and muscle of the skin of koi, with none appearing in the gill.

Diagnosis - Appearance of cysts and presence of characteristic spores within the cysts.

Treatment - No effective treatment is known. Infected fish should be culled. Disinfection of systems which have contained infected stock may prevent spread.

MISCELLANEOUS

Many other fungi have been linked with disease in fish, usually associated with granulomata but also with ulcers and 'tumours', most being only an occasional incidence. Some which have been identified and reported in aquarium fish are mentioned below.

Verticillium piscis - has been seen associated with granulomata in goldfish.

Exophiala pisciphila - has been seen associated with skin lesions in a variety of fish in a marine aquarium.

Aureobasidium sp. - has been seen associated with necrotic lesions in the liver of marine species.

Aphanomyces sp., *Rhizopus* sp., *Phoma* sp. – have all been associated with ulcerative lesions. *Phoma* sp. can also infect the swimbladder.

CHAPTER ELEVEN

BACTERIAL DISEASES

Edward J Branson
Peter J Southgate

GENERAL CONSIDERATIONS

Bacteria are an important cause of disease in fish, and can cause primary or secondary problems. Although there are exceptions, most of the disease causing organisms are aerobic, gram -ve and rod-shaped. Few species can survive above 35°C. Many can exist in a wide range of environmental conditions. None are known to produce spores, so re-infection after cleaning out a tank is unlikely.

As with most systemic disease in fish, generalised bacterial infection is heralded by non-specific signs including lethargy, inappetence, loss of normal colour and fin clamping in those species where this is not normal behaviour. Although some diseases do have characteristic symptoms, some form of bacteriological sampling, followed by identification of the bacteria, is essential for accurate diagnosis. This is usually carried out by examining morphology, staining characteristics and biochemical activity. Other tests which may be available are slide agglutination, immunodiffusion and fluorescent antibody techniques. Histological examination of tissues will occasionally show bacterial colonies within organs, but more commonly will just show general evidence of tissue damage, with or without signs of bacteraemia/toxaemia.

Most fish will have an inherent resistance to bacterial disease, but this resistance will be finite and will be reduced in stressful conditions. Consequently, whereas a low challenge by an infectous organism may be resisted, at some point the infective load may be so great that this ability to resist the disease is overcome. A consequence of this is that once a disease is present within a group of fish, the bacterial loading within the water body can increase to the point where previously resistant fish become susceptible. Because of these facts important aspects of treatment should be the reduction of stress, along with reduction of the infective load in the water by removal of infected fish. These should be carried out in addition to the use of any appropriate chemical treatment.

When a disease causing bacterium has been isolated, the determination of an antibiotic sensitivity pattern for that organism is probably more important than the identification of the organism itself. This is vital, as many importers and suppliers of ornamental fish treat with antibiotics so that there is a strong probability of some antibiotic resistance being present. It should also be remembered that more than one pattern of resistance may be present in bacteria within a given population of fish.

Treatments for diseases discussed in this chapter indicate management procedures and the general classes of chemicals which may be of use in controlling a particular disease (For further information see chapter 21).

CLASSIFICATION OF DISEASE BY PRESENTING SIGNS

Bacterial disease tends to occur in three general forms:
1. acute systemic,
2. superficial and/or ulcerative,
3. chronic granulomatous.

However, few diseases fall entirely within a single category. A list of most of the important disease causing bacteria found in fish is given in the Table 1 (see end of chapter). These bacteria are discussed below, divided into categories according to the type of disease with which they are usually associated.

ACUTE SYSTEMIC DISEASE

Acute systemic disease is usually caused by a primary agent, but can also occur due to secondary invaders in suitable conditions, such as after physical damage or at times of immunosuppression due to severe stress. Generally this type of disease has a sudden onset with loss of appetite. Individuals may show other behavioral changes, and sudden deaths may occur.

After initial entry of the organism there is haematogenous spread and consequent generalised tissue damage. External signs generally appear as erythema and possible petechiation around fin bases, in the grooves on the ventral mandibular surface, around the mouth and vent, and within the operculae. Internally there is usually erythema and petechiation of the internal body surfaces and organs, with some haemorrhages apparent on cut muscle surfaces. The gut may contain blood stained fluid. Organs may be congested, and some degree of ascites is not uncommon. Ascites ('**Dropsy**') and exophthalmos ('**Popeye**') may follow an acute systemic disease, or appear more slowly as a consequence of a more chronic disease. This is thought to be due to the bacteria causing damage to the endocardium and adjacent myocardium, resulting in congestive heart failure. '**Malawi bloat**' in cichlids may be an example of this.

Peracute infections can occur in some diseases, and will often result in sudden death, with no characteristic symptoms.

Due to the systemic nature of this type of disease, bacteria will invariably be found in the kidney. They can be examined in fresh kidney squashes, and can be isolated by inoculation onto appropriate media. Diagnosis can then be achieved by the identification of the causative organism, along with disease signs. Histological examination of tissues will occasionally show bacterial colonies within organs but, more commonly, there may simply be general evidence of a bacteraemia/toxaemia. Clinical findings in all these diseases are as described above unless specified otherwise.

ASSOCIATED ORGANISMS

The most important organisms are:

Motile Aeromonads

These organisms are found world-wide in soil and water (mainly fresh but occasionally marine), and are generally saprophytic. *Aeromonas hydrophila* is the usual pathogen encountered. This is not an obligate pathogen, but can cause disease in stressed fish. Other species may be involved as secondary invaders. All fresh water fish are susceptible and other poikilotherms, such as frogs ('Red Leg'), can be affected. These organisms are commonly seen in carp with Spring Viraemia. Outbreaks are usually related to stress, due to, for example, poor water quality or the fluctuating temperatures seen in the spring. The disease is rare at less than 7-8°C.

Characteristics - Gm -ve, rod shaped, 0.8-1 x 1-3.5 μm, motile with a bipolar (usually single) flagellum. They are aerobic and facultative anaerobes. Some produce brown to red-brown diffusible pigment. They grow well on most laboratory media at 20-22°C.

Disease - Typical signs of an acute systemic disease. Large areas of skin haemorrhage usually occur which may ulcerate.

Diagnosis - Identification of the organism.

Treatment - Remove the primary problem such as stress. Improve water quality to reduce the bacterial load in the water. Antibiotic therapy may be successful.

Pseudomonads

These are ubiquitous organisms, but mostly occur in fresh water. Most are saprophytic, but some are opportunistic pathogens. Disease is usually associated with poor husbandry. All species of fish can be susceptible, and single fish or populations can be affected. A chronic disease is also seen. *Pseudomonas fluorescens* is typical of the group usually associated with disease.

Characteristics - Gm -ve, rod, 0.5-1 x 1.5-4 µm, motile with usually, 1 (sometimes 3) polar flagellum. They are aerobic and many produce diffusible pigments on culture which fluoresce under Ultra-violet light. They grow well on most common laboratory media at 20-25°C.

Disease - Typical acute systemic disease, but with large haemorrhagic skin lesions usually occurring. In the chronic case, the skin lesions may be the only apparent abnormality, and granulomata may form in many tissues.

Diagnosis - Identification of the organism, and the presence of haemorrhagic skin lesions.

Treatment - Improve underlying poor husbandry and reduce stress. Antibiotic therapy may not be of any use due to the usual widespread antibiotic resistance seen in pseudomonads. Surface bactericides may be of use in reducing surface loading and thus minimise the risk of secondary infection.

Vibriosis

This condition can affect fish in all environments, but is usually associated with marine fish. *Vibrio anguillarum* and *V ordalii* are not obligate pathogens, but can be primary pathogens in salt water. Other vibrio species can occur as secondary invaders. Outbreaks are usually stress related, or the organism may gain entry through external injuries, especially in the case of secondary infections. Many species of fish are susceptible.

Characteristics - Gm -ve, *V anguillarum* and *V ordalii* are pleomorphic rods, 0.5 x 1.5-2.5 µm, motile with a single polar flagellum. They are aerobic and grow best on media containing 1.5-3.5% salt at 18-20°C.

Disease - Typical acute systemic disease. Boil-like lesions can occur with *V anguillarum,* leaving deep wounds when they burst. Secondary infection of surface wounds by vibrios can result in shallow skin lesions followed by systemic infection. Due to their ability to produce toxins, some superficial vibrio infections will produce a toxaemia giving the symptoms of an acute bacterial infection. Of course, in this case, no bacteria would be recoverable from the kidneys of affected fish.

Diagnosis - Identification of the organism. Growth on media with added salt and lack of growth in the presence of vibriostats O/129 or Novobiocin is confirmatory.

Treatment - Remove stress in all cases. Improve husbandry in order to prevent wounds through which the bacteria gain entry. Antibiotic therapy of value. Immersion and injectable vaccines are available against *V anguillarum* and *V ordalii,* but are intended primarily for fish farms.

Less common organisms associated with acute systemic disease include:

Edwardsiella

Two species are involved, *Edwardsiella tarda* and *E ictaluri*, which occur in fresh water. Problems are normally seen in cultured fish, especially catfish, but can occur in tropical aquaria. This disease usually occurs in epizootics in conditions of high stress and poor husbandry. *E tarda* is usually seen at temperatures greater than 30°C, *E ictaluri* at 25-30°C.

Characteristics - Gm -ve, rod, 0.5-1 x 1.3-3 μm, motile by peritrichous flagella. They are facultative anaerobes and have an optimum growth temperature of 20-30°C They grow on most common laboratory media, although *E ictaluri* grows quite slowly.

Disease - Typical acute systemic disease in both cases. In addition, foul smelling gas filled lesions appear below the skin with *E tarda,* and these are pathognomonic. *E ictaluri* may show a multi-focal dermatitis and typical '**Hole in the head**' in young catfish.

Diagnosis - Identification of the organism. The presence of gas with *E tarda,* especially in fish kept at around 30°C.

Treatment - Improve underlying poor husbandry and stress, and remove fish showing first signs. Systemic antibiotic treatment may be effective.

Flavobacteriosis

Flavobacterium sp. are common soil and water bacteria (in both fresh and salt water), and are commonly found on fish skin. They are not usually pathogenic, but have been found as opportunist pathogens in injured fish or those in poor condition (usually in fresh water tropical aquaria).

All fish are susceptible in suitable conditions, and the organism may affect single fish or occur in epizootics. This organism is also associated with a chronic granulomatous condition.

Characteristics - Gm -ve, rod shaped, 0.5 x 1-3 μm, non-motile. Most are aerobic with a few facultative anaerobes. Yellow, red, orange or brown pigments are produced in the colonies, but they are not diffusible (i.e: not soluble in the medium).

Pigments usually occur at lower incubation temperatures (10-20°C). These organisms may grow on common laboratory media but, if they do, they may be difficult to sub-culture without special media. Most will not grow below 30°C; some will grow at 37°C.

Disease - Typical acute systemic disease, sometimes accompanied by neurological abnormalities.

Diagnosis - Identification of the organism. Pigmented colonies occur on solid media.

Treatment - Improve underlying problems. Reduce bacterial loading by use of external bactericides and improve water quality. Systemic antibiotic therapy may help.

Streptococcal septicaemia

Streptococcus sp. are ubiquitous organisms which are uncommon pathogens. Outbreaks are usually seen in warm water eg 30°C, and can occur in epizootics. Most species can be affected in the right circumstances.

Characteristics - Gm +ve, oval or spherical, 0.5-1.0 μm in diameter, usually non-motile. They are aerobic, and grow on most common laboratory media, usually in pairs or chains. They may be haemolytic. Incubation temperature should be greater than 20°C.

Disease - Typical acute systemic disease. The kidney may be swollen, and the liver may be dark and congested.

Diagnosis - Identification of bacteria.

Treatment - Improved sanitation and removal of affected fish. Systemic antibiotics may help.

Pasteurellosis

This condition is usually caused by *Pasteurella piscicida*, a marine environmental organism which can produce epizootics in certain circumstances of poor husbandry and poor water quality. A chronic form can occur, called '**pseudotuberculosis**'.

Characteristics - Gm -ve, rod with bipolar staining, 0.5 x 1.5 μm, non-motile. They are aerobic, and grow best on media containing 1.5% salt at 20-25°C. Pleomorphism may occur in older cultures.

Disease - Typical acute septicaemic disease.

Diagnosis - Definitive diagnosis depends on bacterial identification as it resembles non-pigment producing *A salmonicida* in morphology and staining characteristics.

Treatment - Improve husbandry and water quality. Systemic antibiotics may help.

Enteric Red Mouth (ERM)

ERM is seen in fresh water and can affect goldfish and possibly other species. The disease is caused by *Yersinia ruckeri*, a primary and obligate pathogen. Asymptomatic carriers are usually responsible for outbreaks which are normally stress related.

Characteristics - Gm -ve, rod, 1 x 2-3 μm, usually motile with peritrichous flagella but may be non-motile. Aerobic and grows well on most common laboratory media at 22°C.

Disease - Typical acute systemic disease, but in some cases there may be pronounced erythema and haemorrhage, especially around the mouth. Chronic forms can occur with lethargy, skin darkening, sometimes exophthalmos and blindness. The kidneys and spleen may be swollen and the liver is usually pale.

Diagnosis - Identification of the organism. Non-motile forms resemble *A salmonicida*, and motile forms resemble motile aeromonads, vibrios and pseudomonads.

Treatment - Removal of stress and suitable antibiotic therapy. Ideally the disease should be eliminated from the system. Vaccines are available, but are intended primarily for fish farms.

SUPERFICIAL AND/OR ULCERATIVE DISEASE

Some bacteria replicate on the body surface and can directly affect the epithelium resulting in damage to the fins, skin ulceration or gill damage depending on the area affected. Also mechanical lesions may become infected by secondary invaders leading to ulcers.

Skin ulceration can result in systemic invasion by the initiating bacteria, or other secondary invaders. In common with ulcers which are secondary to a systemic disease or mechanical injury, this can result in local and systemic disturbance of the osmoregulatory system. In fresh water, any surface lesion, due to whatever cause, may be quickly invaded by fungus, thus obscuring the underlying problem.

Bacteria associated with superficial and/or ulcerative disease

The most important conditions in this category are:

Carp Erythrodermatitis

Also called '**Goldfish ulcerative disease**' and '**Ulcer disease**'. It can also occur as part of the '**Carp dropsy syndrome**'. This condition is caused by *Aeromonas salmonicida achromogenes*, previously called *Haemophilus piscium*, a variant of the bacterium which causes furunculosis in salmonids. This organism is an obligate pathogen, and carriers can exist. The condition is usually confined to carp. The actual causative organism of furunculosis, *A salmonicida* has occasionally been isolated in cases of 'Ulcer disease'.

Characteristics - Gm -ve, short rod, 1x1.7-2 μm, non-motile. It is aerobic but can be a facultative anaerobe. It is quite slow growing and fastidious, and blood agar is probably the best media to use at an optimum growing temperature of 22°C. No pigments are produced, but the causative agent of furunculosis does produce a brown diffusible pigment.

Disease - This disease is thought to be initiated by the achromogenic aeromonad, ulcers then becoming secondarily invaded by other aeromonads and pseudomonads. The resultant ulcers have a 'punched out' appearance, characteristically with a red centre surrounded by a white rim which itself is surrounded by an erythematous area. A bacterial septicaemia may follow the appearance of these ulcers. Carp erythrodermatitis may be part of a disease complex known as 'Carp dropsy syndrome' or 'Infectious abdominal dropsy', which is associated with Spring Viraemia of Carp caused by *Rhabdovirus carpio* (see chapter 12). The ascites in these cases probably arises due to myocardial damage as discussed in the acute systemic disease section.

'Swimbladder inflammation' is another manifestation of the SVC complex, although it can also be caused by chronic bacterial infection of the swimbladder. This usually results in a characteristic loss of balance due to the intimate association of the swimbladder with the organs of balance.

Diagnosis - Identification of the organism, but this may be difficult due to its fastidious nature. The presence of characteristic ulcers.

Treatment - Oral antibiotic treatment is of limited use, but administration by injection is more successful. Debridement of lesions, followed by the application of a topical antiseptic may help. If *A hydrophila* is involved, then environmental conditions should be improved. Carriers should be removed if possible.

Myxobacterial Disease

The term 'myxobacteria' is the general name often given, not strictly accurately, to bacteria belonging to the family *Cytophagaceae*, also known as '**slime bacteria**'. These bacteria occur as secondary pathogens and opportunistic invaders. Usually only one genus, *Cytophaga*, previously called *Flexibacter*, is involved, but others may occur. These bacteria are common saprophytes in soil and in both fresh and salt water.

Characteristics - Gm-ve, long rods often forming long filaments, 0.5-0.75 x 1.5-30+ μm, motile by gliding. They are aerobic, and all those which are pathogenic are fastidious, requiring specially prepared low nutrient media, such as Cytophaga agar, for culture. *C columnaris* produces a yellow/green pigment in culture.

Disease - Various diseases are attributed to these organisms, usually related to body area affected, but any part of the fish can be susceptible to invasion. Historically, these diseases are classified as follows:

1. Environmental gill disease (Bacterial gill disease)
2. Columnaris disease
3. Cold water disease (Fin rot and Peduncle disease)

These three categories are considered in more detail below:

1. Environmental gill disease

This is often called '**bacterial gill disease**', and is almost always due to environmental problems such as high ammonia levels, leading to invasion of damaged tissue by 'myxobacteria'. This condition is seen throughout the world and can occur in all species, although some are more resistant than others (e.g: carp). The dominant organisms involved are usually *Cytophaga* sp, but others such as pseudomonads and aeromonads may be involved.

Disease - Gill damage, for whatever reason, can result in epithelial hyperplasia. The reduced blood supply in the tissues increases the susceptibility to bacterial invasion, which in turn results in further gill damage until death occurs. Histologically, the degree of gill hyperplasia can be graded according to the thickness of the secondary lamellar epithelium and the amount of fusion between primary and secondary gill lamellae (Post G. 1971 and see Figure 1). The symptoms are typical of any gill disease, with fish gathering at water inlets or 'gasping' at the surface. Operculae may gape revealing red, swollen gills, with excess mucus. White or grey spots may appear on the gills indicating bacterial invasion.

Diagnosis - Fresh gill scrapes may reveal the presence of bacteria and epithelial hyperplasia. Gill changes and the presence of myxobacteria will be visible on histological examination.

Treatment - Identification and removal of the underlying cause of gill damage is vital. Aeration should be used in order to improve oxygen uptake. A surface bactericide can be used to remove bacteria from the gills and also to reduce the bacterial loading in the water, but treatment stress may well precipitate mortality.

2. Columnaris disease

This is also called '**Cotton Wool disease**' and '**Mouth fungus**' due to its appearance on the fish. This latter condition is not uncommon in livebearers, and Black Mollies seem to be particularly susceptible. '**Saddleback disease**' is another synonym, due to the appearance when the dorsal fin is affected. These diseases occur worldwide, and all fresh water fish are susceptible, especially in aquaria. The causative organism is *Cytophaga columnaris*, and the disease itself is almost always a surface infection, chronic to acute. These bacteria are often seen in wet preparations forming 'columns', amorphous masses of bacteria attached to pieces of necrotic host tissue. Seldom does it occur below 10°C, and it can occur as an explosive epidemic above 18°C. Carriers can develop. A similar problem has been seen in salt water, the organism mainly concerned being *C marina*.

Disease - Usually associated with injuries, physiological or nutritional imbalance, or other husbandry problems. Healthy fish are quite resistant to infection. Any part of the body can be affected but often the head is invaded first. The first sign is usually an increase in mucus at the affected area, this developing into the characteristic cotton wool-like growth. This material consists of strands of mucus, necrotic host material and bacteria. Lesions are usually circular, and erythematous areas can occur within them. They may appear yellow or orange due to the pigmentation of the bacteria. Affected fins will usually have necrotic edges. Gills can be affected. Once the bacteria have gained a hold in an infected fish, they will increase the bacterial loading in the water.

Diagnosis - Presence of bacteria in fresh scrapes taken from affected areas. Histological examination of affected tissues will usually show the presence of the bacteria.

Treatment - Improve husbandry to reduce susceptibility of the fish. This will also reduce the bacterial loading in the water, as will the removal of affected fish. Surface bactericides are the best form of treatment, but these must be used early in the disease to be effective since the organism will eventually penetrate the lower layers of the skin where it is more difficult to treat. It is obviously important to differentiate between the cotton wool-like growth of this condition and a fungal infection if the correct treatment is to be given.

3. Cold water disease

This is also called '**fin rot**' when just the fins are affected, and '**peduncle disease**' when affecting the base of the tail. This is a chronic condition, usually seen in cold water from 4-10°C, the causative organism not growing above 12°C. It is seen worldwide and can occur in all fish in the right conditions. The most commonly found organism is *Cytophaga psychrophila*, although other 'myxobacteria', as well as aeromonads and pseudomonads may be involved. A form of peduncle disease may also occur in warm water at temperatures above 25°C.

Disease - Usually secondary to physical damage, physiological or nutritional imbalance, or other husbandry related problem. Once the bacteria have gained entry, they will spread through normal tissue. Usually the condition begins as fin rot and, in the tail, progresses to peduncle disease. The presence of infected fish will increase the bacterial loading in the water and increase the risk of infection in other fish.

Diagnosis - Presence of the bacteria in fresh scrapes from affected areas. Histological examination of affected tissues will often show the presence of the bacteria.

Treatment - Determine underlying primary cause and eliminate it. Surface bactericides will help to kill the bacteria and reduce water loading. Removal of affected fish will also reduce this loading. Systemic antibiotics are usually of little use. If possible, increasing the temperature in cold water fish may help to control infection.

Figure 1: Progressive histological changes seen in gill hyperplasia.

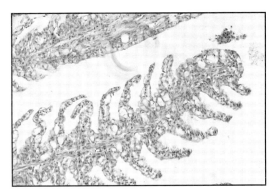

Photo: Ray Butcher   Magnification: X 200

Figure 1a:
Oedema and slight thickening
of secondary lamellar epithelium.

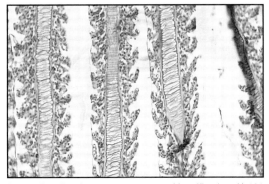

Photo: Ray Butcher   Magnification: X 100

Figure 1b:
More marked thickening of
epithelium but no fusion of lamellae.

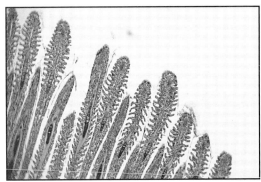

Photo: Ray Butcher   Magnification: X 50

Figure 1c:
Fusion of secondary lamellae
at tips of primary lamellae.

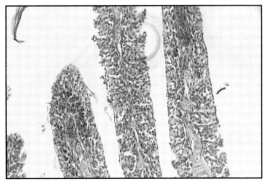

Photo: Ray Butcher   Magnification: X 100

Figure 1d:
Complete fusion of
secondary lamellae.

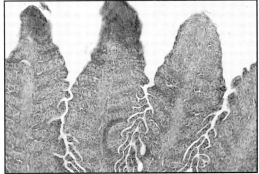

Photo: Ray Butcher   Magnification: X 100

Figure 1e: Complete fusion and
swelling of secondary lamellae
without fusion of primary lamellae

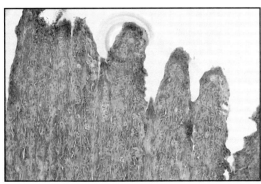

Photo: Ray Butcher   Magnification: X 100

Figure 1f:
Complete fusion of both
secondary and primary lamellae.

A number of superficial and/or ulcerative conditions may occur less commonly. The organisms involved are more often associated with acute systemic disease or chronic granulomatous disease and are dealt with more fully in those sections. These conditions are:

Edwardsiella

Edwardsiella ictaluri can produce a typical '**hole-in-the-head' disease in young catfish**. A multifocal dermatitis of the body wall may also occur. Symptoms of systemic disease are also seen.

Vibriosis

Haemorrhagic skin lesions may ulcerate to reveal underlying musculature. These ulcers may be very deep and even perforate the abdominal wall. Symptoms of acute systemic disease also occur.

Motile aeromonads and pseudomonads

Large haemorrhagic skin lesions may occur, later becoming ulcerated, in a chronic disease. These lesions can also occur associated with an acute systemic disease.

Chronic granulomata

Granulomata forming in the skin or subcutaneous tissues may rupture, thus forming superficial lesions. These may become infected with secondary bacteria or fungus, and do not respond to treatment.

CHRONIC GRANULOMATOUS DISEASE

These diseases involve the production of granulomata within the body of the fish, although if the skin is involved ulceration may follow. The formation of these granulomata is usually very slow, with a consequent insidious onset of clinical symptoms.

Bacteria associated with chronic granulomatous disease

The most important organisms are:

Mycobacteriosis

This is a chronic to sub-acute disease occurring in all kinds of water conditions, especially with overcrowding. It is seen throughout the world and most species are susceptible, as well as other poikilotherms. Oral transmission is most likely, although infection through wounds and via external parasites may be involved. The incubation period is probably 6 weeks or more. All imported fish are potential carriers, and this is the usual method by which the disease is introduced, although other infected poikilotherms may be involved. The most common bacteria involved are *Mycobacterium marinum* in salt water and *M fortuitum* in fresh and brackish water. *M cheloni* has also been isolated. *M marinum* has been associated with human skin problems; the so-called 'swimming pool granuloma' is a hypersensitivity reaction of skin in contact with the organism, but systemic spread does not occur due to the inability of the bacterium to grow at 37°C. *M. fortuitum*, however, will grow at 37°C and has been associated with local abscesses in the extremities of man.

Characteristics - Gm +ve, long straight or slightly curved rods, 0.1-0.7 x 1-10 µm, non-motile. They are acid-fast, and grow on general bacteriological media, although some are more fastidious. *M marinum* is slow growing, the others faster. The optimum growth temperature is 20-30°C.

Disease - There may be no external evidence of disease. Fish may show a number of non-specific signs, such as lethargy and listlessness, some may hide, others may suspend themselves head downward. The appetite is reduced, and emaciation may occur. Skin lesions may result from the rupture of lesions in subcutaneous tissues. Uni- or bilateral exophthalmos may be seen, as may abdominal swelling.

Internally grey/white granulomata of various sizes are seen in all organs, especially the kidney, liver and spleen. These may appear as speckling if many small lesions are present. The lesions tend to be similar in appearance to mammalian tubercles with necrotic caseous centres. The granulomata associated with *M fortuitum* tend to be less focal than those of *M marinum* due to the relative speeds of growth.

Diagnosis - The behaviour of fish, and the presence of acid fast organisms. Characteristic granulomata will be seen on histological examination.

Treatment - No therapy is effective, so elimination of infected fish and disinfection is the only realistic method of control. Detection of carriers is very difficult, although collection of the faeces of individual fish followed by bacterial concentration has been used with some success.

The disease should be avoided by:
1. Quarantine of new fish for at least 2 months
2. Avoidance of overcrowding
3. Not feeding raw, potentially infected food.

Nocardiosis

This condition produces symptoms similar to mycobacteriosis. *Nocardia asteroides* is the organism involved, and this is a common soil organism found worldwide. It is not a common pathogen, but a number of fresh water fish have been infected. The route of infection is not known but is probably via injuries and/or skin damage. The incubation period is long, and carrier fish may be important.

Characteristics - Gm +ve, mycelium-like branched filaments which break into coccoid and bacillus shaped reproductive units, 0.2-0.7 μm diameter. It is acid fast, aerobic and grows well on most laboratory media at 22°C, although the optimum temperature is 37°C.

Disease - As with mycobacteriosis.

Diagnosis - The behaviour of the fish, and the presence of acid fast bacteria distinguished from *Mycobacterium* sp. Characteristic granulomata will be seen on histological examination.

Treatment - There is no known therapy so affected fish should be removed. Morbidity within a population is usually quite low.

A number chronic granulomatous conditions may occur less commonly. The organisms involved in these are more often associated with acute systemic disease and are dealt with more fully in that section. These organisms are:

Flavobacteria

This disease can occur in aquarium fish, typified by the chronic granulomatous condition of Black Mollies. Emaciation, sometimes with exophthalmos has been seen. Internally there is granulomata formation in many organs, especially the liver, similar in appearance to mycobacterial infections.

Pasteurellosis

White 'pseudotubercules' are seen in the liver, kidney and spleen. These usually have a necrotic core surrounded by macrophages. Seen mainly in cultured Yellowtail.

Pseudomonads

Lethargy, exophthalmus and/or ascites are sometimes seen. Focal necrosis throughout the tissues develop into granulomata which appear similar to pasteurellosis lesions.

TABLE 1: Important bacterial fish pathogens

Bacterium	Staining Characteristics	Physical Characteristics	Freshwater or Marine	Clinical features
Motile Aeromonads	Gm - ve	Rod Motile	F & (M)	Acute systemic disease. Haemorrhagic skin lesions which may ulcerate.
Pseudomonads	Gm - ve	Rod Motile	F & (M)	Acute systemic disease. Haemorrhagic skin lesions which may ulcerate. Chronic form with skin lesions and granulomata in many tissues.
Vibrio sp	Gm - ve	Rod Motile	(F) & M	Acute systemic disease with haemorrhagic skin lesions which ulcerate to give deep ulcers. Superficial ulcers may occur with surface infections.
Edwardsiella tarda & E. ictaluri	Gm - ve	Rod Motile	F	Acute systemic disease often with dermal lesions which may ulcerate. Foul smelling gas in *E. tarda* lesions
Flavobacteria sp	Gm - ve	Rod Non-motile	F&M	Acute systemic disease or granulomatous condition
Streptococcus sp	Gm + ve	Coccoid Non-motile	F & M	Acute systemic disease
Pasteurella piscicida	Gm - ve	Rod Non-motile	(F) & M	Acute systemic disease or granulomatous condition - 'psuedotuberculosis'
Yersinia ruckeri	Gm - ve	Rod, Motile or Non-motile	F	Acute systemic disease, sometimes with skin haemorrhage around the mouth.
Aeromonas salmonicida achromogenes	Gm - ve	Rod Non-motile	F	Haemorrhagic skin ulcers often followed by acute systemic disease.
Cytophaga sp (Flexibacter)	Gm - ve	Rod to filament Motile by gliding	F & M	Skin, grill and fin lesions.
Mycobacterium sp	Gm + ve Acid fast	Rod Non-motile	F & M	Tubercular lesions.
Nocardia asteroides	Gm + ve Acid fast	Branching filaments Non-motile	F & (M)	Granulomata

F - Freshwater, M - Marine, ( ) - unusual occurrence

CHAPTER TWELVE

VIRAL DISEASES

Peter J Southgate
Edward J Branson

Although numerous viral agents and diseases of possible viral aetiology have been described in fish, only a small number are, at present, of importance in ornamental fish.

CARP POX

Carp pox results in an epidermal hyperplasia and is found in a number of carp species. It is thought to be the result of infection with a possible herpes virus, and is described more fully in chapter 14.

SPRING VIRAEMIA OF CARP

Introduction - Spring Viraemia of Carp (SVC) is undoubtedly the most important virus disease of ornamental, as well as wild and farmed carp. It is probably also of some importance in other Cyprinids.

SVC is often included as a component of the complex of diseases known as the 'carp dropsy syndrome', or 'infectious dropsy'. Although the syndrome can be divided into two major disease entities, SVC and carp erythrodermatitis (CE - discussed under bacterial diseases), the picture is complicated in that fish with SVC may well be suffering secondary or even primary bacterial infection. The carp dropsy syndrome will be discussed more fully under bacterial diseases.

A notifiable disease - SVC has recently become far more important in the U.K. following numerous outbreaks of infection in 1988. Until then, although endemic in several European countries, particularly those with intensive carp culture, only four isolated cases had been identified within Great Britain. In 1988 the infection was confirmed in 36 sites in England and Wales. The majority of these outbreaks were confined to fisheries but some involved ornamental fish dealers and hobbyists. The occurrence of the outbreaks was thought to be related to the import of ornamental fish from France.

The disease is notifiable under the diseases of fish act 1937 (as amended), and anyone suspecting an outbreak should notify the appropriate Ministry laboratory (see chapter 23).

The disease - In infected sites, the disease usually occurs as water temperatures begin to rise in the Spring, frequently following a cold, stressful winter when the fish have been crowded or suffered physical damage. Fish which have not encountered the infection previously are susceptible at any time, but clinical acute disease will only occur when the water temperatures are sufficiently high (i.e. above 8°C), and then significant losses can occur.

Clinical signs of the infection include lethargy and darkening of the skin. The fish can exhibit signs of respiratory distress and loss of balance. Abdominal distention (dropsy) and exophthalmos (popeye) are usually pronounced and petechial haemorrhaging of the gills and skin may also be present. Internal visceral haemorrhages, and the presence of sero-sanguinous fluid within the abdominal cavity are the most frequently reported findings, and there may also be a fibrinous peritonitis. Secondary bacterial septicaemia is often identified.

Treatment and Control - Although there is no treatment for the disease itself, it may be possible to reduce the extent of secondary bacterial infection with the use of antibiotics, providing treatment is initiated early in the course of the infection. Surviving fish appear to have a strong immunity to re-infection, but may well become persistent carriers. Because of the highly infectious nature of the virus, and the severe consequences of spread of the disease, a slaughter/disinfection policy may be the most appropriate control measure. It is extremely important that great care is taken over the disinfection of equipment, clothing etc. used in infected areas to prevent virus being carried to non-infected stocks.

If SVC is identified, a movement order is placed on the affected site. The movement of live fish from the site is then prohibited until the order is lifted. Control of this disease obviously lies with the careful observance of disinfection procedures in infected areas, the prohibition of imported infected fish, suitable quarantine measures, and the prevention of movement of fish from infected to non-infected areas. The possibility of non-carp species acting as asymptomatic carriers will always make control difficult, a problem applying to many fish diseases.

SWIMBLADDER INFLAMMATION (SBI)

Introduction - Swim-bladder inflammation (SBI) has been described as a component of the carp dropsy syndrome, and is thought to be a separate entity from SVC, although the aetiological agent is thought to be identical to the virus causing SVC.

The disease - Usually affecting Cyprinids in their first summer, the disease is manifested by abdominal distension, exophthalmus and loss of balance. In more acute cases, darkening of the skin and loss of balance may be the only observed symptoms prior to death.

On post-mortem, pathology is usually restricted to degenerative changes of the swimbladder, with congestion, haemorrhage and frequently sloughing of necrotic epithelium into the lumen. Often only one chamber of the swimbladder is affected.

Spread of infection appears to be rapid in affected populations of fish, leading to high levels of mortality. Secondary bacterial infection may be present.

Treatment and Control - As with SVC, the control relies on the isolation of affected stocks and the prevention of spread of infection to uninfected fish. Antibiotic therapy may assist in reducing the incidence of secondary bacterial infection.

LYMPHOCYSTIS

Introduction - This viral infection has been described in many species of fresh-water and marine fish. The cause has been identified as a DNA virus, and there is some evidence that a group of closely related viruses, each with some species specificity, is involved.

The disease - The disease is chronic in nature and results in the development of small circumscribed skin nodules (frequently described as pearl-like). The single or multiple lesions can most often be seen on the skin or fins of the fish, but can also be found on the gills, inside the mouth, or within the abdominal cavity. Infection of connective tissue fibrocytes or fibroblasts with the virus causes the infected cell to enlarge to many times it's original size. This results in the formation of macroscopically visible nodules (lymphocysts), which continue to increase in size over the following months, sometimes reaching 2cm in diameter. The time-scale of development of the lesions varies with the temperature and species involved, but it is normally within the range of one to three months. When many lymphocysts are present, the skin can take on a 'sandpaper-like' appearance. Eventually an inflammatory reaction surrounds the lymphocysts which then undergo necrosis and slough, leaving an intact epidermis. The condition, although unsightly, is rarely fatal.

Infection is thought to take place through skin abrasions, and is more severe under conditions where fish are crowded or undergo frequent handling. The dissemination occurs when the lesions rupture or slough.

Treatment and Control - There is no treatment, and although full recovery is usual, recurrence of the lesions can occur. It is therefore preferable to obtain fish from known disease-free stocks.

CICHLID VIRUS (RAMIREZ DWARF VIRUS)

Introduction - This virus has not yet been isolated, but has been seen on electron microscopic studies, and is thought to be responsible for acute disease in the South American tropical fish *Apistogramma ramirezi*, imported as an aquarium fish into the USA.
Other imported cichlids may well be affected by the virus, and quarantine is advisable.

The disease - The disease has a course of 3-4 weeks, and a mortality of between 40-80% in affected stocks. Clinical symptoms of the disease are inappetence, pallor, respiratory distress and haemorrhages of the skin and iris. As the disease progresses degenerative changes of the eye occur. Internally, the gut is empty, the spleen enlarged, and all the viscera appear pale. The pathology consists of general degenerative changes of the spleen, intestine, liver, kidney, pancreas and eyes.

GENERAL CONSIDERATIONS - OTHER POSSIBLE VIRAL DISEASES

It is very likely that other viral agents are associated with disease in ornamental fish, and these may well be identified in the future as virological capabilities and investigations progress. In general, provided adequate precautions are taken with regard to selection of stock, quarantine, isolation of possibly infected animals and awareness of the need to prevent the spread of infectious agents, problems associated with virus disease should be minimised.

A second important consideration regarding virus disease in fish is the accidental importation of viruses which may not affect the fish being imported, but pose a threat to other native or cultured species. A particular case would be the salmonid viruses, **Viral Haemorrhagic Septicaemia (VHS)** and **Infectious Haemopoietic Necrosis (IHN)**, which at present are not found in the UK. There is a risk that these viruses could be imported with fish, or water, from Europe or the USA, and find their way into the UK wild or cultured salmonids, particularly where carp and salmonids are held within the same facility. This emphasises the need for strict control on imported stocks and the need for adequate quarantine.

CHAPTER THIRTEEN

TOXINS

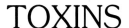

Peter J Southgate
Edward J Branson

GENERAL CONSIDERATIONS

The range of elements and compounds, either natural or man-made, which are toxic to fish is vast. The toxic effects of metabolic products of fish and other naturally occurring substances has been covered under environmental aspects (chapter 7). This chapter is concerned with the effects of exogenous substances introduced into the water, either by natural processes, or by the action of man.

The quality of the water supply to fish holding facilities can vary considerably, and depends very much on geographic location, the nature of the water supply, and the treatment processes to which the water is exposed. 'Natural' supplies of water (i.e: rainwater, borehole, spring or river water), can be of very good quality, but there are potential hazards from each of these supplies, and if contemplating using these as a source of water checks should be carried out to assess the suitability.

PROBLEMS OF NATURAL WATER SUPPLIES

Rainwater

Dissolved gases (Sulphur dioxide SO_2, carbon dioxide CO_2, and hydrogen sulphide H_2S), produce a low pH (acid rain). There may also be dissolved and suspended organic and inorganic material from atmospheric pollution.

Borehole

Water from boreholes may show extremes of pH. There may be unacceptably high levels of dissolved heavy metals, as well as high levels of suspended solids.

Spring or River water

There may be a low pH, particularly in areas prone to acid rain and/or forestry run off. There may be the additional problem of the acidified water dissolving metals from the river bed (especially if the rock has no buffering capacity, e.g: granite). This is a particular problem with aluminium, which is frequently present in high quantities in acid waters and is at its most toxic at a pH around 5.

High levels of suspended solids may be present. There is also a danger of the transmission of infectious agents when using spring or river water.

Domestic water supply

The vast majority of people will use the domestic water supply and in general this is of a consistently good quality. There will be regional variations in quality and it is always preferable to obtain a basic water quality analysis before using a supply for fish - remember that a water authority is only responsible for supplying water fit for human consumption, and this may not always be suitable for fish.

With domestic water supplies, dissolved metals (copper, lead, aluminium) may be a problem, particularly in older supplies and the levels of these should be checked.

Chlorine is another frequent problem. All water used for fish should be allowed to stand for at least 24 hours, preferably with aeration, to allow any dissolved chlorine to dissipate. An alternative to this would be to fit an activated carbon filter to the supply which may also help to remove other contaminants.

Alum is sometimes added to the water supply as a flocculent to remove colour and suspended material from the water, particularly in 'peaty' supplies. Alum may enter the domestic supply as a flush and is directly toxic to fish.

CLINICAL SIGNS ASSOCIATED WITH THE PRESENCE OF TOXINS

Many of the symptoms exhibited by fish are common to a wide range of toxic substances.

Death

Acute poisoning (e.g: following a flush of chlorine through the system), will frequently result in a complete fish kill with the fish showing little gross abnormality (infectious agents will very rarely cause a 100% mortality of fish).

Respiratory distress

Sublethal levels of several categories of toxins have a damaging effect on the gills or respiratory physiology. This will cause the fish to exhibit signs of respiratory distress (i.e: 'gasping' at the surface of the water, hyperventilation, crowding at water inlets).

Behavioural changes

Avoidance behaviour may be seen if there is room for the fish to move away from the toxic substance. This may take the form of jumping or abnormal and erratic swimming.

Water imbalance

Sub-acute or chronic exposure to a toxin may result in impairment of the ability of the fish to control water balance, and this may manifest itself as abdominal swelling ('dropsy'), scale lifting and exophthalmos ('popeye').

Chronic effects

Chronic exposure to some toxins, particularly heavy metals, can result in retarded growth, loss of reproductive capability and deformity.

Other symptoms will be discussed under specific toxins.

CATEGORIES OF TOXIC AGENTS

There are five main groups of substances which are potentially toxic to ornamental fish.

Metals	Aluminium, copper, lead, iron, zinc, cadmium
Gases	Chlorine is the principal exogenous gas which is toxic to fish. Other toxic gases (eg: H_2S) may be found, but are invariably the result of natural processes within the pond or aquarium (see chapter 7.).
Organic compounds	Petrochemicals, wood preservatives, paints etc.
Biocides	Pesticides, herbicides, algicides etc.
Therapeutic agents	Formalin, malachite green, antibiotics

TOXIC METALS

Introduction

Many metals have been implicated in causing death and pathological effects in fish. Those most commonly cited as potentially harmful are aluminium, copper, cadmium, iron, zinc and lead. Lead, iron, and zinc may leach into the water from older domestic systems, and it is important that any water which has been in such a system for some time is flushed through before any is used for fish. Copper could be a potential hazard of newer systems, and it is advisable to flush the system before drawing water for use.

Water abstracted from springs or boreholes which passes through metal-bearing rock, or comes into contact with industrial outfalls, may contain toxic levels of metals.

There are many variables which could make a metal more or less toxic. The pH, hardness, the presence of organic material or other elements can dramatically affect the toxic effect of the metal. In general a low pH will lead to a higher solubility of the metal in the water and therefore a more toxic effect. There are, however, exceptions to this. In water of pH above 7, iron will be precipitated as a colloid on the gills of fish and block gaseous exchange. In addition, although the aluminium ion is probably most toxic at a pH around 5, at a pH of 8 and above the alumate ion will cause a toxic effect.

Hardness will tend to reduce the toxic effect of a metal, and hence higher levels of a metal will be tolerated in hard water.

The presence of organic material in the water will tend to reduce the toxic effect of a metal by adsorbing a quantity of the element while, in contrast to this, additional metals and other chemicals in the water may have an additive or synergistic effect. All these factors must be taken into account when assessing a situation or data for evidence of metal toxicity.

Clinical signs and pathological effect of metal toxicity

The toxic effects of metals can range from the highly acute, sudden death of an entire stock, to a slow chronic pathology resulting in growth depression, deformities and low grade mortalities. Sublethal effects include respiratory distress and water imbalance.

Species and age will have a bearing on the effect of exposure to toxic metals. Young fish will be more susceptible to the lethal effects of acute exposure and are more likely to show developmental abnormalities caused by exposure to sub-lethal levels. Raised levels of mortalities in eggs are found in cases of metal toxicity, and developmental abnormalities are more likely in fish hatched from surviving eggs.

The principal organs to be affected by metal toxicity are the gills, the kidney and the liver, although other tissues may more rarely be involved.

Gills

As the gill can only react in a limited number of ways to the presence of an insult, the clinical symptoms seen, and the pathology detected, are very similar for a wide range of toxins and water quality problems. The following may therefore be applied to many of the factors causing gill damage discussed in this manual.

In acute metal toxicity, gill damage may be the only pathology detected. Histological examination will usually show necrotic and hypertrophic changes of the gill epithelium with a possible increase in mucus activity (this may be detected grossly, as may a similar increase in skin mucus).

Sub-acute to chronic exposure results in proliferative changes (hyperplasia) of the gill epithelium which may be detected on examination of fresh gill preparations. These hyperplastic changes reduce the respiratory capabilities of the fish and give rise to the respiratory distress seen particularly at times of reduced oxygen availability.

With a continuing or frequent exposure to the toxin, there may well be a combination of acute and chronic effects, and a fish with chronically damaged gills will be more susceptible to the acute effects of a toxin or other water quality problem. The damaged gills are also very prone to secondary bacterial and fungal infections, and this underlying gill pathology must be borne in mind if considering any treatment for such secondary infections, as the therapeutic agents may themselves be damaging to the gills.

Kidney

Absorption of a toxic metal is very likely to cause necrosis of the haemopoietic and excretory tissue of the kidney. Hydropic swelling and necrosis of the kidney tubules is a frequently described finding.In surviving fish, this will result in fibrosis and loss of tubular tissue with a consequent reduction in excretory ability and the symptoms of water imbalance described above.

Liver

Toxic metals can be directly damaging to the liver giving rise to a patchy necrosis and perivascular fibrosis in surviving fish. Patchy liver necrosis may also be a consequence of anoxia or hypoxia resulting from the presence of any chronic gill damage.

Safe levels of metals

As indicated above there are many variables affecting the toxicity of metals and it is therefore difficult to give accurate values for levels of metals which would be considered safe in acute or chronic situations. The following table is a guide, but species and age susceptibility, and water quality parameters must be taken into account.

Solubility and toxic levels will vary greatly with pH, hardness and possible antagonistic/synergistic effect of other substances in the water. A very large safety margin (by a factor of at least 100) should be allowed for acceptable levels of these metals under normal circumstances.

Levels of metals generally considered toxic to fish (All values in mg per litre)	
Copper	3.0
Aluminium	0.3
Cadmium	0.1
Iron	0.3 - 10.0 (Very variable)
Lead	1.0
Manganese	2.0
Chromium	5.0
Mercury	1.0
Zinc	1.0

TOXIC GASES

Chlorine

Chlorine is the only toxic gas to be considered in this section. The gas is directly toxic to the gills of the fish and will cause acute necrosis of the gill epithelium. Sub-lethal exposure often results in necrosis of the tips of the secondary lamellae with adhesion or fusion of adjacent lamellae. Chronic exposure causes localised or general hyperplastic change of the gill epithelium. The toxic effect varies with the species concerned and toxicity is reduced somewhat if the organic loading of the water is high. Symptoms of chlorine toxicity are restricted to distress, respiratory failure and death.

TOXIC ORGANIC COMPOUNDS

The range of organic compounds which are toxic to fish is vast, but under normal circumstances there will be few occasions when ornamental fish are likely to be exposed to these compounds. In the aquarium, the only means of exposure is by the accidental introduction of the material into the water by the aquarist. Many wood preservatives and treatments are toxic, and so any wood introduced into the aquarium (e.g: ornamental bog oak) must have been treated with a non-toxic compound. Many of the polishes, paints and D.I.Y. materials used in the house are also toxic, and should never be used in the vicinity of aquaria.

The risk of organic poisoning to pond fish is very dependent on the source of the water. Spring supplies are susceptible to pollution episodes upstream, and also run-off and discharges from agriculture and industry. Borehole water is less at risk, but there is always the possibility of pollutants finding their way into the water table. Domestic supplies should pose a very much smaller risk.

The use of toxic organic compounds in the vicinity of garden ponds, or in their construction, or the accidental spillage of these compounds is the most frequently encountered form of organic poisoning in pond fish.

Examples of toxic organic compounds

A thorough discussion of organic compounds toxic to fish, their effect and detection, is outside the scope of this manual. The following is a short list of compounds which can have a lethal or a variety of sub-lethal effects.

    Phenolic compounds
    Benzene
    Oils
    Grease
    Polychlorinated biphenols (PCBs)
    Detergents

Sources of these include petrochemical, wood and paper processing, and many other industries.

Clinical signs

These substances can be toxic in a variety of ways. Oils can coat the surface of the fish and cause asphyxiation. They can be directly toxic to the gills and, when absorbed, can cause damage to many internal tissues. Phenols and benzene can have similar effects. PCBs can accumulate in fish tissue and cause physiological effects such as a reduction in reproductive capacity and possible immunosuppression. Certain compounds in all categories have been implicated as carcinogens.

Clinical symptoms of organic toxicity will obviously be very variable, but will include distress and avoidance behaviour, respiratory failure and death. Sub-lethal effects may include osmotic imbalance, blindness, haemorrhage, anaemia, skin lesions, loss of balance, poor growth and loss of reproductive ability.

Diagnosis will be based very much on suspicion and detection of a pollution event.

BIOCIDES (pesticides, herbicides, molluscicides etc.)

The majority of these compounds are directly toxic and, unless it is a preparation formulated for use in a fish holding facility and used correctly, contamination of aquaria and ponds from domestic use of these compounds should be avoided. The major risk to fish health from pesticides is run-off from agriculture, and sometimes industry, contaminating the water supply. The effect can be lethal or sub-lethal, many of the compounds having a cumulative effect in the body of the fish.

Important categories of pesticides in relation to their toxic effects on fish are the organochlorines (OCs) and organophosphates (OPs). In addition to these are the 'natural' pesticides, such as pyrethrum, and their synthetic analogues which are also toxic.

Several examples of the organochlorine group, which includes DDT and dieldrin, have been banned, or are subject to restricted use in the UK. As the OCs are fat soluble, they can accumulate in fat depots, and be released when the fat is metabolised. There can, therefore, be a significant delay from the fish having absorbed the toxin and the development of pathological effects. The toxic effects of OCs include central nervous damage and necrotic change of the liver and kidney.

Organophosphates act as cholinesterase inhibitors and are used as pesticides for the treatment of crustacean and other ectoparasites in fish, as well as being used extensively as pesticides in agriculture, horticulture, domestically and in industry. They can be directly toxic to fish, causing paralysis and death if overdosed, or if present in sufficient quantities in water sources. Although rapidly broken down in the water, they can have a cumulative effect from frequent exposure, reducing overall brain and tissue cholinesterase levels. This reduction in cholinesterases has been implicated in poor growth and performance and in the development of spinal deformities. If OP poisoning is suspected, brain cholinesterase estimation may help in the diagnosis.

Pyrethrum is a natural insecticide obtained from dried chrysanthemum flowers. It is toxic and should be used with care in the vicinity of aquaria and ponds. Little is recorded of its toxic effect and detection.

Rotenone is another natural insecticide of plant origin which has been used for many years, and is lethal to fish. Indeed it is used as an effective piscicide to eliminate unwanted fish from bodies of water. Clinical symptoms of rotenone poisoning are those of asphyxiation and, if suspected, detection is dependent on the demonstration of rotenone in the water.

As a general rule domestic and veterinary insecticides,including sprays and slow-release fly strips, should never be used near aquaria or fishponds.

TOXICITY OF THERAPEUTIC AGENTS

By their very nature the majority of therapeutic compounds used to treat fish are biocidal in their activity and can have a toxic effect on the fish if used at levels other than those recommended for a particular set of conditions or if the fish is compromised in any other way (e.g: by intercurrent disease or gill pathology). It is extremely important, when contemplating a treatment, that water quality parameters, and the condition of the fish themselves, are taken into account before commencing with the treatment.

Many of the compounds used for bath treatment, such as formalin, malachite green, chloramine-Tx and benzalkonium chloride (BAC), have a damaging effect on the gills and, although this should be minimal when the treatment is used as recommended, if overdosed or if gill pathology is already present, significant damage can be caused to the gills. This damage could result in death, or render the fish more susceptible to secondary infection and further gill pathology. As the toxic effect of some treatment compounds is dependent on the pH or hardness of the water (e.g: chloramine T and benzalkonium chloride are more toxic in soft water), it is essential to assess at least these two parameters before calculating a dose rate.

A basic assessment of gill condition should also be attempted before treating and, although this may be difficult, obvious signs of respiratory distress or the presence of high numbers of gill parasites would suggest caution in carrying out a treatment.

A test treatment on a small number of fish should always be carried out when possible.

Formalin

Formalin is a reducing agent and, as well as being directly toxic to the gills, it will lower the level of oxygen in the water (this may also apply to other treatment compounds). It is therefore important to use oxygenation or aeration during a treatment to maintain levels of dissolved oxygen.

Paraformaldehyde, recognised as white crystals, can form in formaldehyde solutions. This is toxic to fish, and any formalin used in fish treatment must be free from this substance.

Malachite green

Malachite green is toxic to the gills and blocks the enzymes of respiration in the fish (oxygenation may not therefore be of great assistance in cases of overdose). This compound will also accumulate within tissues and can result in liver and gill pathology following repeated treatments.

Anaesthetic agents

All anaesthetics are toxic, and can be lethal if overdosed or if the health of the fish is compromised in any way.

Organophosphorus compounds

These are used as pesticides in fish, and their toxic effects are discussed above.

Disinfectants

The majority of disinfectants are highly toxic, and should never be used in the presence of fish.

Anti-bacterial agents

The antibiotic and antibacterial agents used in fish can also have toxic effects whether given in feed or parenterally. Sulphonamides, and potentiated sulphonamides, can be a particular problem in marine fish, where crystallisation in the kidney and consequent renal damage is a possibility following prolonged use. Oxytetracycline has been shown to be hepatotoxic following intra peritoneal injection and, as with other therapeutic agents, it is important that the suggested dose rates are adhered to.

General considerations

There are several other reported adverse or toxic effects of therapeutic agents, including the possibility of malachite green causing developmental abnormalities when used to treat fish eggs.

Certain antibiotics may cause suppression of erythropoiesis and the immune response. It must also be borne in mind that several of these compounds have been implicated as possible carcinogens or having other adverse effects on man.

MISCELLANEOUS TOXINS

Heavy metal contamination, and the other toxic effects of feed, are discussed in chapter 15.

Cases of malicious poisoning have been encountered in fisheries, cyanide being the most commonly employed agent, but it is hoped that this would be a much less likely event with ornamental fish

THE INVESTIGATION OF A CASE INVOLVING A POSSIBLE TOXIC AGENT

Diagnosis

The wide range of possible toxic agents and the generally non-specific nature of the clinical signs and pathology encountered makes conclusive diagnosis extremely difficult. In many cases there may be a suspicion of the presence of a toxin (i.e: a history of a pollution episode, an obvious deterioration in water quality, or the use of potentially toxic agents in the vicinity of an aquarium or a pond). This will generally apply to acute cases. Chronic exposure to a toxin will have a far more insidious effect and will be less easy to identify.

Clinical symptoms may well indicate the presence of a water-borne toxin. A total fish kill points strongly to a toxin (infectious agents will rarely cause 100% mortality), although factors such as a sudden fall in oxygen levels might also produce this. Avoidance behaviour, abnormal swimming movements and respiratory distress may indicate the presence of a sublethal level of a toxin.

Laboratory analysis

Water analysis, histopathology and toxicological analysis of fish tissues can all be used in investigating the presence of a toxic agent.

Water samples should be taken as soon as a water quality problem is suspected. If a serious pollution episode is suspected, the local water authority should be notified. If there is a possibility of litigation, or if malicious poisoning is suspected, duplicate samples of the water should be obtained, and these should be sealed and signed in the presence of an independent witness.

Obtaining water samples

The following points should be considered:

1) The container must be chemically clean (it may be possible to obtain these from a laboratory). At the very least they should be rinsed several times in distilled water (not forgetting the cap) and also rinsed at least five times in the water to be analysed.

2) The containers should be of inert plastic with plastic tops. Glass bottles and metal tops should be avoided.

3) At least a litre of water should be collected, and the container filled to the top, excluding all air.

4) The sample should be kept cool, and forwarded rapidly to the laboratory. If the sample has to be stored, it should be filtered and deep frozen

Other samples

Samples for histopathological analysis should be obtained from moribund or very freshly dead fish (see chapter 20). Tissue samples, usually muscle and liver, can be taken for toxicological analysis.

These should be deep frozen immediately after sampling. In the case of suspected organophosphate (OP) poisoning, the brain should be removed and frozen. Tissue samples for toxicology should then be forwarded on ice (dry ice preferably) to the laboratory, having given prior warning of their despatch.

The three areas of laboratory investigation which can be used for detecting the presence of a toxic agent are thus:

> Water analysis (raised levels of the toxin in the water)
> Pathology (specific pathology present indicative of a toxin)
> Toxicology (raised levels of the toxic agent in tissues)

The following table gives an indication of the comparative value of these three techniques when applied to different categories of toxin:

Value of tests for categories of toxin			
(++ = valuable; + = may be of some value; - = no value)			
Category of toxin	**Water analysis**	**Pathology**	**Toxicology**
Metals	++	++ (gill liver kidney)	++
Gases	-	++ (gill)	-
Toxic organics	- *	-	- *
Biocides	+ **	-	+ **
Therapeutic compounds	-	+	+

*   It is difficult to analyse for organics unless the identity of the agent is suspected.

**   It is possible to analyse water or fish tissue for the majorcategories of biocides (for suspected OP poisoning the acetyl cholinesterase activity of the brain tissue is assessed).

In cases of cyanide poisoning, it is usually necessary to analyse tissue samples for the presence of this compound, pathology and water analysis being usually of no value

ACTION IN CASES INVOLVING A POSSIBLE TOXIC AGENT

1)   Remove source of toxin if known

2)   Obtain water samples

3)   Remove dead fish, but keep them frozen in case of insurance or other investigation

4)   Flush fresh water through the system or carry out water changes (preferably with 'seasoned' water)

5)   Ensure adequate oxygenation

6) Stop feeding the fish

7) Obtain samples for histopathology and toxicology from moribund or very freshly dead fish.

8) Notify insurers if a claim is likely.

9) Notify the water authority if pollution or poisoning issuspected.

10) Notify the laboratory of any samples being taken.

11) Monitor the situation for prolonged effects or secondary disease.

CHAPTER FOURTEEN

NEOPLASIA

Peter J Southgate
Edward J Branson

GENERAL CONSIDERATIONS

As with terrestrial animals, neoplasia, with some specific exceptions, becomes more common with the increasing age of the individual. The relative longevity of some pet fish inevitably means that tumours will be encountered in some of the older, no doubt highly-prized, specimens.

There is no reason to doubt that all fish tissues are capable of neoplastic transformation, and tumours of the majority of organs have been recorded at some time, in a variety of species. Tumours of the skin are the most frequently reported, but this may simply be a consequence of their ease of observation.

Neoplasms are usually classified by the cellular origin of the tumour, but for the purposes of this manual, classification will be based upon whether the tumour is visible on the surface of the fish (i.e: there may be some possibility of surgical removal), or whether the tumour is internal (i.e: surgical intervention is unlikely).

The degree of invasiveness of skin tumours varies from a simple area of hyperplasia, through non-invasive true papillomata, to very invasive carcinomata penetrating the underlying tissues. Although surgical removal of these lesions is a relatively straightforward procedure, the success of surgery and possibility of recurrence will very much depend on the invasive properties of the neoplasm.

SURFACE TUMOURS

Papillomata

These are common in many species of fresh water and marine fish. The tumour is benign, of epithelial cell origin, and can vary in form from a slightly raised area of hyperplastic epidermis to very obvious papillary projections of the skin. There are often multiple tumours present.

Carp pox

Carp pox is frequently classified as a neoplasm, although strictly it is a virus-induced hyperplasia of the epidermis found in most cultured species of carp. The disease occurs as multiple raised shiny white/grey lesions on the body and fins of the fish. The lesions, which are discrete areas of epidermal hyperplasia, often have the appearance of drops of candle wax on the fish and can usually be removed quite easily. As carp pox is of viral aetiology it can occur as an epidemic in fish ponds, and it is not unusual to see many fish affected. The disease is seasonal and self-limiting, the lesions developing in spring and disappearing as temperatures drop in late summer.

Immunity to the infection is thought not to be very strong, and it is possible for the disease to recur in following years. There is some evidence that surgical removal evokes a stronger immune response.

Lymphocystis

This is a virus disease, principally of marine fish, causing small, pearl-like lesions on the skin. This condition has occasionally been mistakenly identified as neoplasia, and will be considered in more detail in chapter 12.

Neurofibroma/Fibroma

These are relatively frequent tumours found in goldfish, presenting as a single, or multiple, subcutaneous mass causing a swelling beneath the skin of the body wall. Surgical removal has been attempted but, because of the deep and invasive nature of the lesion, is unlikely to be successful.

Melanoma

Tumours of the pigment cells of the skin are not infrequent, melanomata being the most common. An example is the melanoma found in a hybrid of the platy-swordtail, resulting in a raised black area of the skin (occasionally the eye) with extensive local invasion

Miscellaneous sites

Apart from melanomata found in several species and occasional neural tumours, ocular neoplasia is rare. Similarly, tumours of the gill tissue are infrequently encountered.

INTERNAL TUMOURS

Although intra-abdominal masses may be suspected in a fish with a long-standing abdominal swelling, the presence of a tumour is usually only diagnosed on post-mortem. Exploratory laparotomies are a very infrequently performed procedure in fish.

Tumours of the visceral organs

Tumours of the liver, pancreas, kidney, gonads, swim-bladder and gastro-intestinal tract have all been described in a variety of species of ornamental fish. The majority take the form of single or multiple masses within the abdominal cavity and frequently become extremely large.

Tumours of mesenchymal origin

Neoplasia of tissues of mesenchymal origin (myomata, osteomata, lipomata etc.) are relatively common in fish. In addition to the fibroma in goldfish mentioned above, fibromata and fibrosarcomata may be seen as swellings of the body wall covered by normal epidermis in many fish species.

Tumors of haemopoietic tissue

Neoplasia of the haemopoietic tissue has been described. Lymphosarcoma often takes the form of an ulcerating, subcutaneous lesion, with metastases to other organs.

EMBRYONAL TUMOURS

Nephroblastoma

This has occasionally been identified in young fish.

Teratoma

This embryonal tumour is found mainly in tropical fish. Most often seen in guppies, this tumour is composed of mixed tissue types, and usually takes the form of a prominent ventral abdominal swelling.

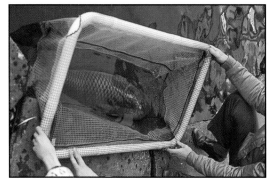

Photo: Ray Butcher

Plate 1:
Slime disease in a carp – giving
a blue-grey sheen to the skin.

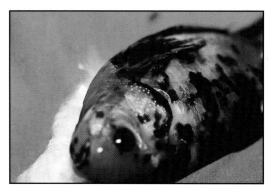

Photo: Ray Butcher

Plate 2:
White spot on the gill cover
of a koi carp, due to *Ichthyophthirius*
***multifiliis* infection.**

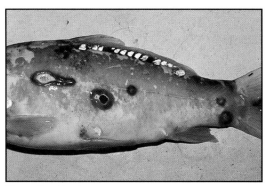

Photo: Ray Butcher

Plate 3:
Ulcerated granulomatous lesions in
a koi following *Lernaea* infestation.

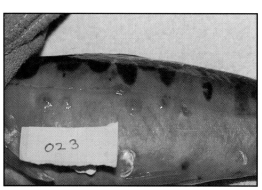

Photo: Ray Butcher

Plate 4:
Multiple skin nodules in koi
due to *Dermocystidium* infection.

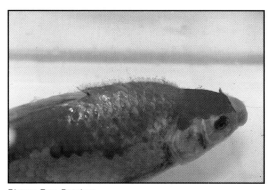

Photo: Ray Butcher

Plate 5:
***Saprolegnia* hyphae on the**
dorsal surface of a koi.

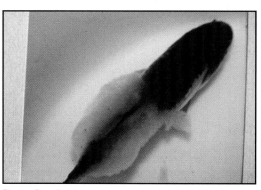

Photo: Ray Butcher

Plate 6:
Extensive growth of *Saprolegnia*
on a goldfish.

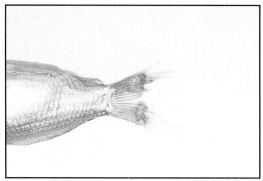

Photo: Ray Butcher

Plate 7:
Fin rot due to infection by
***Cytophaga* sp. (*Flexibacter* sp.).**

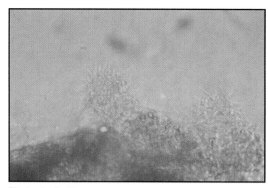

Photo: Lydia Brown

Plate 8:
Microscopical appearance of
***Cytophaga* sp. (*Flexibacter* sp.).**

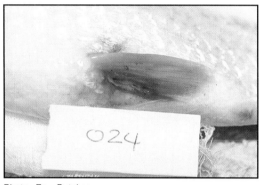

Photo: Ray Butcher

Plate 9:
Hyperaemia of fins as a sequel to
systemic bacterial infection.

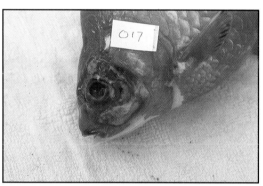

Photo: Ray Butcher

Plate 10:
Erosion of the tissues of the head
of a goldfish due to *Aeromonas* sp.
infection.

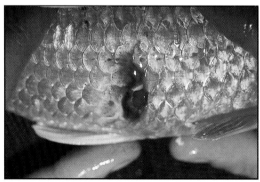

Photo: Ray Butcher

Plate 11:
Localised ulceration of the
skin with scale loss.

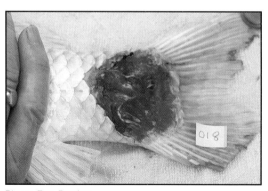

Photo: Ray Butcher

Plate 12:
Extensive ulceration at the
root of the tail in a koi.

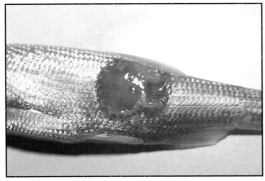

Plate 13:
Granulating ulcer in an orfe
(*Leuciscus idus*).

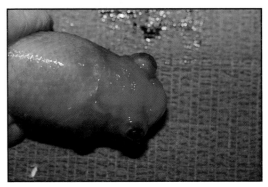

Plate 14:
Bilateral exophthalmos
in a goldfish.

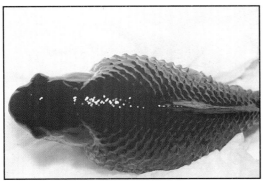

Plate 15:
"Pine-Cone" effect due to raising of
scales as a sequel to dropsy.

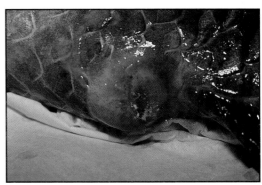

Plate 16:
Oedema of the vent as a sequel to
generalised bacterial infection.

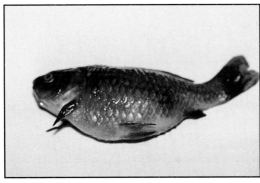

Plate 17:
Generalised septicaemia in a goldfish
showing haemorrhages on the skin.

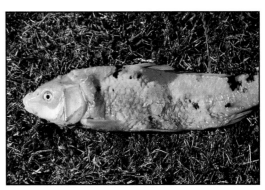

Plate 18:
Emmaciation in a koi resulting from
generalised *Mycobacterium* sp. infection

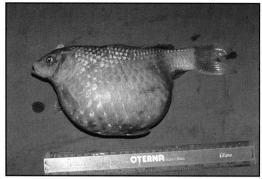

Photo: Ray Butcher

Plate 19:
"Dropsy" – gross enlargement
of the abdomen.

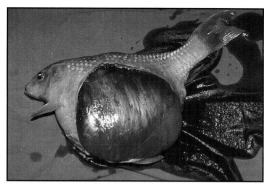

Photo: Ray Butcher

Plate 20:
Removal of the body wall muscle
from the fish in Plate 19 to reveal
a fluid-filled abdominal cavity.

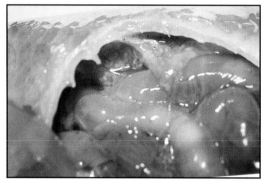

Photo: Ray Butcher

Plate 21:
Oedematous changes in the
bowel and viscera.

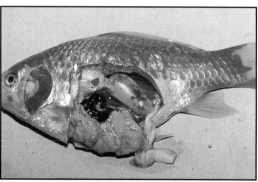

Photo: Ray Butcher

Plate 22:
Septicaemia and haemorrhages on the
viscera including the swimbladder.

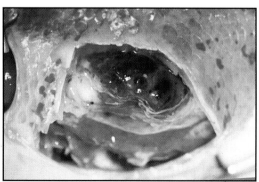

Photo: Ray Butcher

Plate 23:
Septicaemia with swelling and
haemorrhage of the kidney and
haemorrhages on other viscera.

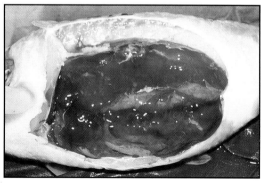

Photo: Ray Butcher

Plate 24:
Oedema and haemorrhages throughout
abdominal cavity. *Mycobacterium* **sp.**
isolated from liver and kidney.

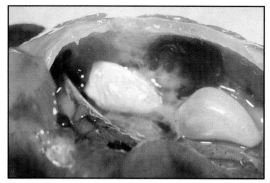

Photo: Ray Butcher

Plate 25:
Collapse of anterior portion
of the swimbladder in a koi.

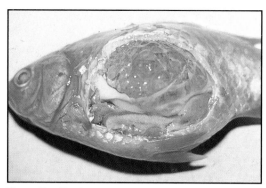

Photo: Ray Butcher

Plate 26:
Polycystic kidney
in a goldfish.

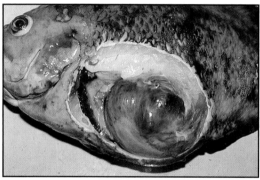

Photo: Ray Butcher

Plate 27:
Large cyst associated with a
Microsporidian infection of the
kidney in an Oscar (*Astronotus* sp.).

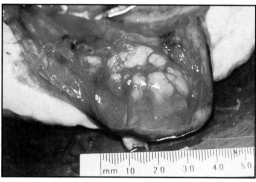

Photo: Ray Butcher

Plate 28:
Adenocarcinoma of the
pancreas in a koi.

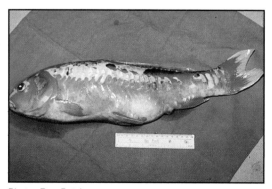

Photo: Ray Butcher

Plate 29:
Discrete swelling in the posterior
abdomen of a koi (as opposed to
generalised swelling seen in dropsy).

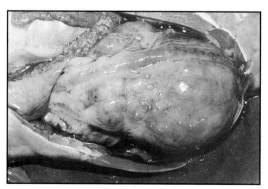

Photo: Ray Butcher

Plate 30:
Exposure of the abdominal cavity of
the fish in Plate 29, showing an
adenocarcinoma of the bowel.

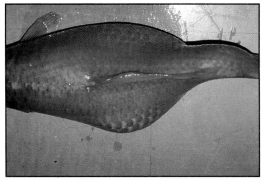

Photo: Ray Butcher

Plate 31:
Asymmetrical swelling due to a fibroma
in the muscle of the body wall.

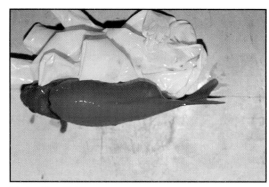

Photo: Ray Butcher

Plate 32:
Granuloma in the body wall of a
goldfish due to *Mycobacterium* sp.

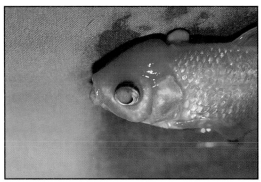

Photo: Ray Butcher

Plate 33:
Papillomata on the neck
and cornea of a goldfish.

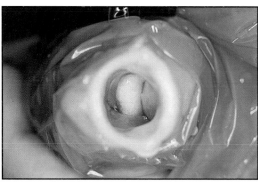

Photo: Ray Butcher

Plate 34:
Intra-oral papilloma in a
koi (removed surgically).

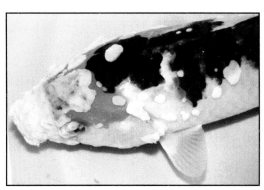

Photo: Ray Butcher

Plate 35:

"Candle Wax" lesions
due to Carp Pox.

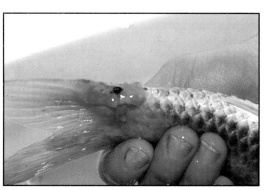

Photo: Ray Butcher

Plate 36:

Invasive fibrosarcoma at the
root of the tail in a koi.

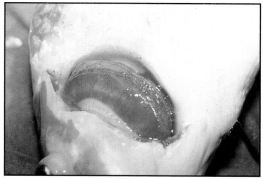

Photo: Ray Butcher

Plate 37:
Gross appearance of the gills
showing excessive mucus and
swelling of the lamellae.

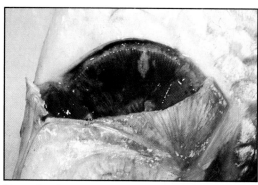

Photo: Ray Butcher

Plate 38:
Gross appearance of the gills
showing necrotic lesions
of bacterial gill disease.

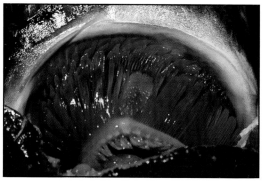

Photo: Ray Butcher

Plate 39:
Gross appearance of the gills
showing discrete lesion of
Branchiomycosis in a koi.

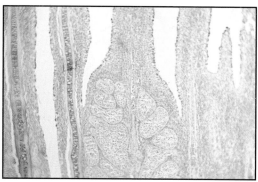

Photo: Ray Butcher   Magnification: X 100

Plate 40:
Histological section of the gill
stained with H&E showing cysts
due to *Henneguya* sp. infection.

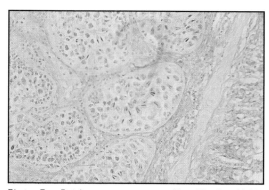

Photo: Ray Butcher   Magnification: X 200

Plate 41:
Section as in Plate 40, stained with
Giemsa to show characteristic polar
bodies of *Henneguya* sp.

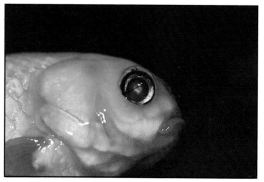

Photo: Ray Butcher

Plate 42:

Cataract in a goldfish –
aetiology unknown

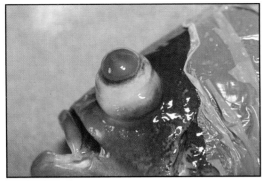

Photo: Ray Butcher

Plate 43:
Unilateral exophthalmos in an
Oscar (*Astronotus* sp.), due to
multiple retrobulbar granulomata
(? *Nocardia* sp. infection).

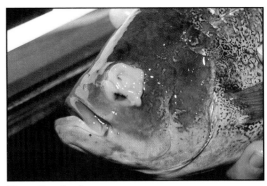

Photo: Ray Butcher

Plate 44:
Post-operative packing of
the orbit from Plate 43
with Orabase.

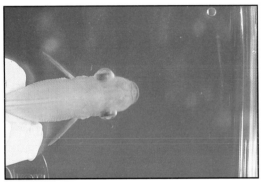

Photo: Professor Gratzek

Plate 45:
Gas bubble disease
showing in both eyes.

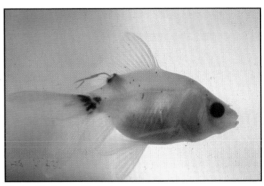

Photo: Professor Gratzek

Plate 46:
Anchor worm (*Lernaea* sp.) attached
to the dorsal surface of a goldfish.

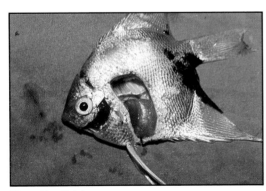

Photo: Ray Butcher

Plate 47:
Exposure of the abdominal cavity of an
angel fish to illustrate species variation
in size and distribution of the viscera.

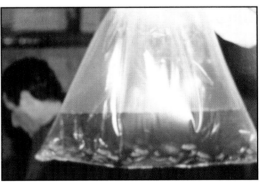

Photo: Ray Butcher

Plate 48:
Tropical fish imports - densely stocked
poly bags, oxygenated and transported
in insulated polystyrene boxes.

CHAPTER FIFTEEN

NUTRITIONAL DISEASES

Peter J Southgate
Edward J Branson

GENERAL CONSIDERATIONS

In the majority of cases commercial diets appear to satisfy the nutritional requirements of ornamental fish, and nutritional disease is a rarely diagnosed problem. There are, however, a number of situations where nutritional disease may manifest itself.

1. Insufficient food given, resulting in total nutritional deficiency (starvation). This leads to poor growth, poor survival, an increased susceptibility to disease and a loss in reproductive capacity.

2. The provision of an imbalanced diet due to the feeding of one particular foodstuff (e.g: meat), to the exclusion of others. This may lead to deficiencies in certain essential nutrients.

3. Idiosyncratic needs or feeding behaviour of certain species. Many diets may not adequately meet the needs of particular species of fish, and reference should be made to specialist texts. Special diets, or supplementation of commercial diets, may be necessary in these cases.

4. Poorly formulated diets. This is unlikely to occur with the good quality control of commercially prepared diets.

5. Use of poorly stored, or out of date diets. This may lead to oxidation of fats and the degeneration of vitamins, etc.

6. The presence of toxic factors in the diet, either through contamination, or from the presence of toxic factors within a constituent of the diet. Again, with good quality control and formulation this is unlikely to occur.

GENERAL PROBLEMS

Starvation

Starvation can result from the inadequate provision of food, for example, when the number of fish present is underestimated, or when insufficient food is given in order to avoid polluting the water. Competition between fish, whether through size disparity or different feeding behaviour between species, will frequently result in inadequate nutrition of certain individuals. This is a particular problem in community tanks, where it is essential that all fish have access to the food.

Starvation may also occur if fish are presented with food of inappropriate physical characteristics, such as size, texture etc., or if fish with idiosyncratic requirements are given the wrong diet. This is a common problem when weaning and raising young fish. Signs of starvation may also occur if there is a lack of essential dietary factors, for example certain amino acids, fatty acids and vitamins etc. Growth, viability and breeding potential, etc., will all be limited by the levels of these factors present.

All the above factors should be considered when presented with a possible nutritional deficiency. It is particularly important that an optimum plane of nutrition is maintained in breeding groups to ensure the fecundity of the brood fish, and the viability of the eggs/fry.

Constipation

The faeces are normally short, and are dropped quickly from the body. Retention and trailing of faeces (often with entrapped air bubbles) indicates that the fish is constipated. Constipation can be the result of overfeeding on dry feed, and is sometimes thought to occur when old, poorly stored food is given. The retained faeces can affect swim bladder function and cause problems with balance. A change in diet to live food and possibly a higher fibre (vegetable) intake should improve the problem. With-holding normal food, and purging with a small piece of bread soaked in halibut oil has also been advocated, and a small rise in water temperature may also help.

SPECIFIC NUTRITIONAL PATHOLOGIES

In contrast to starvation, where there is a total nutritional deficiency, several pathological conditions have been associated with specific nutritional deficiency or toxicity. The principal pathologies, and possible causes are detailed in Table 1.,and, although none are unique to a nutritional imbalance, the latter should be included in the differential diagnosis if any of these conditions are identified.

The list in Table 1 is by no means exhaustive, and many other nutritional factors have been implicated in one or more of the conditions.

Many other pathologies and abnormalities have been described in relation to nutritional imbalance (anorexia, poor growth, poor pigmentation, exophthalmia etc.), but these findings are too non-specific, being found in a wide variety of nutritional and non-nutritional disease, to be of assistance in pinpointing a specific nutritional problem.

IMBALANCES OF SPECIFIC NUTRITIONAL COMPONENTS

Proteins

The protein requirement of fish is high and the majority of natural feeds eaten by fish are protein rich. Commercial diets are also high in protein, and it is unlikely that a protein deficiency will occur.

It is possible, however, for deficiencies of one or more of the essential amino acids (EAA) to occur for the following reasons;

1)   The use of a poorly formulated diet containing components lacking in certain EAAs (particularly plant proteins) or from antagonisms in diets containing an excess of some EAAs. The latter may result in the preferential uptake of some to the exclusion of others.

2)   Leaching of amino acids into the water. This has been reported to occur with frozen, or freeze-dried natural feeds.

3)   Heat or chemical treatment during manufacture causing the breakdown of some amino acids.

Deficiency of one or more of the EAAs will result in retarded growth, and possible loss of breeding potential. More specifically, methionine or tryptophan deficiency is known to cause cataract. Tryptophan deficiency has been implicated in vertebral deformity in a number of species and has also been associated with fin erosion and susceptibility to Myxobacterial disease.

Table 1: Specific nutritional pathologies

Pathological condition	Possible cause	
Cataract	Zinc	deficiency
	Copper	deficiency
	Selenium	deficiency
	Tryptophan	deficiency
	Methionine	deficiency
	Riboflavin	deficiency
	Vitamin A	deficiency
	Excessive dietary calcium	
	Choline	toxicity
Vertebral deformity	Phosphorus	deficiency
	Tryptophan	deficiency
	Vitamin C	deficiency
	Cadmium	toxicity
	Lead	toxicity
Fatty degeneration of the liver	Fatty acid	deficiency
	Choline	deficiency
	Excessive dietary fat	
	Oxidised fat toxicity	
Fin erosion and susceptibility to Myxobacterial disease	Fatty acid	deficiency
	Tryptophan	deficiency
	Riboflavin	deficiency
	Vitamin C	deficiency
Skin/fin haemorrhages	General vitamin deficiencies	

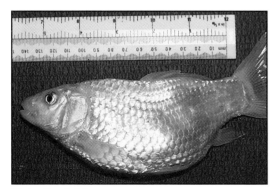

Photo: Ray Butcher

Figure 1
Vertebral deformity in Carp
(Gross appearance)

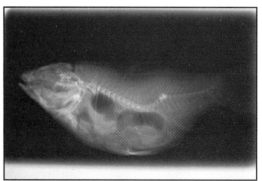

Photo: Ray Butcher

Figure 2
Vertebral deformity
in Carp

Carbohydrate

An intake of excess carbohydrate in ornamental fish is reported to cause degenerative change and excessive glycogen deposition in the liver. In a large number of fish species, the liver is an important fat storage organ, and naturally contains very high levels of fat within the hepatocytes. It is therefore relatively easy with an excessive intake of carbohydrate, to overburden the liver and cause degenerative changes which lead to a deterioration in the health of the fish.

Lipids

As with carbohydrate, an excessive intake of dietary fat may lead to fatty degeneration of the liver. Deficiency of any one or more essential fatty acids will result in poor growth and decreased viability/breeding potential. Fatty degeneration of the liver, and an increased susceptibility to finrot and Myxobacterial infections has also been reported in some species fed a diet deficient in essential fatty acids.

Much of the lipid contained in fish diets is composed of polyunsaturated fatty acids which, without adequate antioxidant protection, are very prone to oxidation (rancidity), resulting in fatty degeneration/ceroidosis of the liver caused by the intake of these oxidised fats. The usual causes of the diets becoming rancid are poor storage of food in a damp, warm environment, the use of out of date food, or the lack or loss of antioxidant. Vitamin E has a very important role in protecting fats from oxidation, and rancidity readily occurs in vitamin E deficient diets (vitamin C also has a role as an antioxidant).

The various products of fat oxidation (peroxides, ketones etc.) can have several toxic effects and also interfere with the nutritional value of other dietary components. The major pathological effect, however, is to cause severe degenerative changes in the liver.

There is frequently an associated anaemia due to the toxic effects of the oxidised fats on the haemopoietic system. Cardiac and skeletal muscle pathology may also be found, most likely due to the deficiency of vitamin E in the diet.

The combination of this hepatocellular degeneration, anaemia and muscle pathology has a profound effect on the health and survival of the fish. Depending on the extent of the damage, there may be a relatively rapid onset of mortalities over a few days with few preceding symptoms, but more frequently there is a chronic sequence of events, with some or all of the following symptoms:

> Inappetence
> Lethargy
> Ascites
> Popeye
> Pallor
> Nervous behaviour
> Increasing mortalities

On gross post mortem there is frequently pallor of the gills, fluid retention in the abdomen and an enlarged, greasy, friable liver, often bronze or bright orange in colour (note that the livers of normal ornamental fish are often fatty and orange in colour). A definitive diagnosis is dependent on the histopathology and feed analysis. Blood analysis for anaemia and liver damage may be of assistance.

Recovery will depend very much on the extent of liver damage. In the early stages there should be a good response to a normal diet, but recovery is doubtful in cases where there is extensive liver destruction.

Vitamins

Vitamin deficiencies can arise from poor formulation, processing or storage of feeds. Loss of water soluble vitamins can readily occur through leaching into the water. Very high losses can occur (especially of vit C) if the feed remains uneaten in the water for any length of time. It is unlikely that commercial diets for ornamental fish will be deficient in vitamins, although some authorities believe that most pet fish are suffering sub-clinical vitamin deficiency, and advocate the use of a multivitamin supplement.

Many abnormalities have been identified with deficiency of specific vitamins. Several of these are general findings, such as anorexia and reduced growth. Some of the more specific disorders related to vitamin deficiency, are detailed in Table 2.

Table 2: Symptoms of specific vitamin deficiencies

Vitamin Deficiency	Disorder
Riboflavin	Cataract Fin erosion and susceptibility to Myxobacterial disease
Pantothenic acid	Generalised hyperplasia of the gill leading to fusion of the gill filaments (nutritional gill disease)
Pyridoxin	Nervous disorders, hyperexcitability
B12	Anaemia
Choline	Fatty degeneration of the liver
Ascorbic acid	Skeletal (particularly vertebral) deformities. Fin erosion and susceptibility to myxobacterial infection
Vitamin A	Cataract/corneal opacity
Vitamin E	Fatty liver/ceroidosis. Muscle pathology

Deficiency of a number of different vitamins, or 'general vitamin deficiency', has been described as a cause of fin and skin haemorrhages.

Vitamin toxicity

Although toxicity of choline has been described as a cause of cataract in fish, it is very unlikely that toxic levels of vitamins would be found in ornamental diets. Vitamin toxicity has only been encountered with experimental diets and will not be considered here.

Minerals

Mineral deficiencies/toxicities have been little studied in fish. Those mineral deficiencies which have been looked at invariably produced the usual sign of reduced growth. Some of the more specific pathologies related to mineral deficiencies are detailed in Table 3.

Table 3: Specific symptoms of mineral deficiencies

Mineral	Deficiency States
Zinc	Cataract (NB high calcium levels in the diet will compete with zinc and may lead to cataract)
Iron	Anaemia
Iodine	Goitre
Phosphorus	Skeletal abnormalities

Mineral Toxicity States

As mentioned above, high levels of calcium in the diet (e.g: those containing high levels of fish/bone meal), although not toxic per se, may compete with other elements, such as phosphorus, iron, manganese and zinc to cause an apparent deficiency. These include cataract, anaemia and skeletal deformity.

Heavy metal contamination of dietary constituents can occur, particularly if by-products from other commercial processes are used in the formulation of the diets. The effect of these metals in the diet is likely to be similar to that seen when they are water-borne (see chapter 13).

Toxicity of certain heavy metals, particularly lead and cadmium, has been identified as a cause of vertebral abnormalities in several species of fish.

Other nutritional toxins

There are several classes of substances which are potentially toxic if present in the diet as contaminants.

1. Therapeutic agents - (see chapter 13)
2. Biological agents - algal, fungal, bacterial toxins eg aflatoxin, botulinum toxin
3. Organic agents - biocides, hydrocarbons

Very little work has been carried out on the toxic effect of most of these compounds on ornamental fish. It is likely that they would be identified only if there was strong circumstantial evidence indicating their presence.

Pathogens

It is possible that parasites, bacteria or viruses may be transmitted in the food, particularly if live food is given. Various helminth parasites are frequently carried as their larval forms in some invertebrates which may be used as live food, and bacterial and viral pathogens of fish have also been isolated from a number of live foods.

Bacterial species, such as *Mycobacterium* sp., and fungal spores may be present as contaminants in feeds, and may cause a chronic systemic infection in fish when these feeds are ingested.

Commercial diets are unlikely to be contaminated with viable pathogens, but live feeds, or feeds containing fresh fish products pose a real threat. To a certain extent this may be avoided by various pre-treatments of the food, but this will not guarantee the absence of pathogens.

INVESTIGATING NUTRITIONAL DISEASE

It is often difficult to identify the presence of a nutritional disease, as many of the associated symptoms (eg: reduced growth etc.) are of a very non-specific and often extremely chronic nature.

The history of poor growth, poor survival, low fecundity and any of the more specific symptoms outlined in this chapter should, however, alert the practitioner to the presence of a possible nutritional problem. Histopathology of affected fish will also assist in the identification of a nutritional imbalance, although in many cases it will not be possible from this to identify specific nutritional deficiencies/toxicities.

If a nutritional pathology has not developed beyond the point of recovery, a change in diet, or a nutritional supplement may bring about a great improvement in the condition of the fish and further investigation may not be necessary. A more detailed investigation into the cause of a probable nutritional imbalance can be very difficult, time-consuming and costly.

Important Considerations

The following factors are important to consider:

1. The species involved, and their particular nutritional requirements.
2. The clinical history - time of onset of problem
                          - general condition of fish
                          - specific symptoms
                          - intercurrent disease
3. Nutritional history. As nutritional disease may take many weeks to manifest itself, it will be necessary to obtain details of feeding over an extended period of time. Particular attention should be paid to the freshness and storage of the food.
4. Histopathology. This is frequently the most useful method of determining the presence of nutritional disease and, wherever possible, tissue samples of affected fish should be taken for histopathology whenever nutritional disease is suspected. Other standard laboratory procedures, such as bacteriology, may also be necessary to rule out the presence of other disease processes.
5. Feed analysis.

Based on the clinical and pathological findings, it may be possible to identify more specifically the nutritional imbalance involved. It may then be possible to carry out analysis of the food to confirm the presence of a deficiency or toxicity.

Problems associated with Feed Analysis

For several reasons, however, the analysis of the feed can be very unrewarding:

1. As stated above, nutritional disease can have a very chronic progress and it is quite possible that deficiencies occurring in the diet may not manifest themselves as clinical phenomena for many weeks, by which time the fish may well be on a different diet. Analysis of the present diet will not therefore give any meaningful results. It will frequently be necessary to examine previous batches of food, and for this reason it is useful to retain frozen samples of previous batches of feed.
2. For meaningful analysis it is necessary to retain relatively large quantities of the feed and, unless dealing with a situation where large volumes of food are consumed, it is often impossible to do this.
3. There may be no clear indication of the dietary imbalance involved, and although a nutritional disease may be suspected, it would not be possible to analyse the food for all the possible specific elements.
4. Information and data on the nutritional requirements of many species is very limited and, unless there is extreme deficiency or excess, it is often very difficult to interpret results of food analysis

CHAPTER SIXTEEN

GENERAL APPROACH

Ray L Butcher
Lydia A Brown

Fish clients frequently complain that veterinarians are not interested in their aquatic pets. There may, therefore, be a degree of prejudice with respect to ones ability to diagnose and treat fish diseases. It is important to begin by asking the correct questions and be aware that a great deal of self medication may already have occurred. More than with any other companion animal, the environment of the fish can be the primary factor in the development of disease. Since fish live in a "bacterial soup", it follows that all healthy fish in a contaminated aquarium or pond are at risk, and so measures must be taken to quickly eradicate the disease and restore a healthy environment.

Home visit / Examination at the surgery

Ideally home visits should be made, as this permits the examination of the fish in its normal environment, as well as all the other in-contact fish. Further to this, it allows a thorough appraisal of the management and environmental conditions, and avoids the additional stress associated with transporting the fish.

The disadvantage is that the time spent on such visits needs to be charged for realistically, and the resultant fee may be unacceptable to some aquarists. Others, however, much prefer this professional approach to their problems and are quite willing to pay the appropriate fee.

The less desirable alternative is for the client to bring the fish to the surgery. This should be done with the fish in plenty of aquarium/pond water. The bag in which it is placed should be insulated so as to maintain a constant temperature, and preferably a second container of aquarium/pond water should be brought in case anaesthesia or treatment is required. Potentially, the level of fees may again be a problem, and so it is wise to discuss the likely cost of the procedure prior to the consultation. In any event, a full clinical examination including anaesthesia will be a time consuming procedure, and so is best not arranged during the middle of a busy surgery.

Where visits are made to a number of different premises, one should always consider the risk of accidentally transferring organisms and hence spreading disease. Thought should therefore be given to adequate protective clothing, personal hygiene and a disinfection protocol.

Client records

It is important to record information relating to the basic management of the system, including the type of filtration system, normal water quality parameters and the aquarist's husbandry practices (eg: frequency of water quality testing). Whenever possible, the environment of the fish should be examined when the fish are healthy, and this ideally should involve a visit to the pond system or fish room before a problem arises. It is extremely useful to have a mental picture of what the system looks like, and how it functions, under normal conditions.

Items which are important to consider are given in Table 1.

Table 1: A checklist of management factors to be recorded

Fish	-	species
	-	numbers / size
	-	frequency of introducing new fish
	-	quarantine procedure
Plants	-	types
	-	frequency of introducing new plants
	-	quarantine / pretreatment procedure
Feeding	-	type of food
	-	frequency of feeding
	-	storage
Pond/aquarium	-	volume of water
	-	surface area
	-	source of water
	-	how long established
	-	frequency and method of cleaning
	-	siting within room or garden
Water circulation	-	pumps - types and capacity
	-	water changes - proportion / frequency / source
	-	average loss through leaks / evaporation
	-	waterfalls / fountains / airstones
	-	material used in pipe manufacture
Filtration	-	types
	-	capacity
	-	how long installed
	-	frequency and method of cleaning
	-	u/v filters - size and position
Heating	-	types
	-	thermostats / monitoring
Lighting	-	natural
	-	artificial - types of tube
Water quality	-	parameters tested
	-	frequency of testing
Routine treatments	-	medications used
	-	dosage
	-	frequency

The collection of this basic information can easily be achieved by the client filling in a questionnaire - in effect registering with the practice as a "fish client". In addition, the client should be encouraged to inform the practice of any changes in his system, and to keep his own records relating to treatments given, disease problems and fatalities etc.

Such records are not only an invaluable aid to investigating a subsequent disease outbreak, but are also essential if the practice is considering dispensing prophylactic medications to these clients.

Client education

As with the investigation of any disease problem, the process is made much easier by the active cooperation and understanding between the Veterinarian and the client. It is important to make the client aware of the range of diagnostic procedures available, but also that these may only be possible if suitable material is submitted. Perhaps the commonest problem is the presentation of dead, decaying fish for post-mortem examination. Only *very* fresh material is of any value, such that it is preferable for a client to submit a dying fish to the surgery for euthanasia and *immediate* post-mortem. Similarly, if there is a problem in a large batch of fish, it might be preferable to sacrifice a representative sample for analysis. Such methods would be common in intensive farming systems, but may not always be accepted by fish clients, who may know all their fish as individuals, and may not like to give up on a dying fish in case a miracle cure occurs.

The Veterinarian must always remember that ornamental fish are truly companion animals, and the emotional feelings of some aquarists mirror those of dog and cat owning clients.

The investigation of a disease problem

Always approach the problem in a standard manner. The steps taken are summarised in Table 2.

Taking a good history is obviously very important, and care should be taken to ensure that it reflects what the client has actually seen, rather than his own interpretation of the problem based on popular pet-fish disease books.

The remainder of this section of the manual looks in more detail at items (b) to (d) referred to in Table 2.

"First Aid"

If there is a delay in the time of examination, or if a specific diagnosis requires waiting for the results of laboratory tests, then the following procedures can be utilised as a first aid measure to reduce stress.

1. Isolation of affected fish.
   Remove them from the system and keep in quarantine. (N.B. Koi appear to like company and some people suggest that a small koi be placed in quarantine with a larger sick one if it is to be isolated).

2. Reduce or even eliminate feeding until the cause of the problem is established.

3. Improve aeration / oxygenation if possible.

4. Check filters.

5. Reduce stocking density if possible

6. Check water quality parameters and repeat daily as necessary

7. Perform regular partial water changes

Table 2: Basic steps for investigating a disease problem

a) History

    1. An appraisal of the underlying system and management (as above)

    2. History of current problem:
- Numbers / species of fish affected
- timescale
- presenting symptoms
- mortalities

    3. Possible changes in management acting as a trigger
- filter changes
- pond / aquarium cleaning
- changes in feeding regime
- introduction of new fish / quarantine
- faulty heating, lighting, or pumping equipment
- power cuts

    4. Possible environmental changes acting as a trigger
- fluctuating temperatures
- algal blooms
- predators (cats, herons)
- sudden leaf fall

    5. Self medication
- compounds used (Many aquarium remedies do not have active ingredients listed but it is essential to try to discover the basic composition of the compound).
- dosage and treatment protocol

    6. Possible exposure to toxins
- aerosols, solvents, weed killers etc.

b) Examination of the environment / water testing

c) Examination of the fish

    1. Examination of all in-contact fish
    2. Examination of affected fish within pond / aquarium
    3. Clinical examination of fish out of the water

d) Laboratory examination

    1. Post-Mortem procedure
    2. Further laboratory tests

CHAPTER SEVENTEEN

EXAMINATION OF THE ENVIRONMENT

Lydia A Brown
Ray L Butcher

GENERAL WATER QUALITY

Aquarists check water quality to a variable degree. Those who check regularly are least likely to have problems since they will catch signs of disease early on. The corollary to this is that these same clients are also the most likely to self-medicate at the first sign of a problem. If the problem persists, it may become extremely difficult for a diagnosis to be made, since all the original signs may be masked by these remedies.

As a general rule of thumb, a good aquarist will check water quality parameters on a weekly basis. Maintenance of filter media will occur as necessary, probably on a monthly basis. With respect to water quality, it is not uncommon to find aquarists attempting to keep fish from totally different aquatic environments in the same tank, resulting in stress to those species least suited to the system. A good encyclopaedia of fish is an absolute necessity to discover the aquatic environment from which the fish has originally come, and hence its requirements.

Water quality parameters which are within the normal range but bordering on toxic levels can themselves be stressful and induce disease in the system. What is important as a basic rule is that sudden environmental changes can kill, and even transient changes, which then rapidly return to normal (for example a power cut inducing change of water temperature and reduced oxygen for a short period), can be lethal.

Water quality parameters to be measured

The water quality parameters that are routinely measured are given in Table 1, but the reader is referred to Chapter 2 for a full discussion on the subject. It must be stressed that the tolerated levels of these parameters vary greatly with different fish species. They are also closely inter-related, such that a variation in one may affect the levels of the others (e.g. the level of unionised ammonia is dependant on both the pH and the temperature). Great care is thus needed in the interpretation of test results, and the levels given in Table 1 can be little more than a broad guide.

Table 1: Water Quality Parameters – Guide to Tolerated Ranges.
(all values in parts per million, ppm)

	Tropical Marine	Fresh Water
Total ammonia nitrogen (TAN)	<0.1	<0.1
Unionised ammonia	<0.02	<0.03
Nitrite	<0.01	<0.5
Nitrate	<20.0	<50.0
Dissolved oxygen	>5.0	>6.0
Chlorine	Negligible	Negligible

Other parameters that should be measured are:

> pH
> Alkalinity
> Hardness
> Salinity
> Copper levels

Individual fish species have adapted to different ranges of these parameters, such that generalisations about tolerated ranges are not possible.

The tolerated levels of other toxic agents (e.g. heavy metals) together with the procedure for their analysis are discussed in Chapter 13.

Testing equipment

The level of total ammonia nitrogen (i.e. the sum of that present as free ammonia and as the ammonium ion) can be measured using standard test kits. The appropriate reagents are added to a fixed volume of the water to be tested and a colour change produced. The value of TAN is obtained by comparing the colour produced to that of a series of standards.

Similar test kits are available for measuring pH, nitrite, nitrate, chlorine, alkalinity, hardness and copper. These test kits are obtainable from:

1. Hach test kits
   Supplied by Norlab Instruments
   Site 9, Kirkhill Industrial Estate
   Dyce, Aberdeen.
   Tel (0224) 724849

2. New Technology Ltd
   Unit 13, Branbridge Industrial Estate
   East Peckham
   Tonbridge, Kent, TN12 5HF
   Tel (0622) 871387

3. Interpet Ltd
   Interpet House
   Vincent Lane
   Dorking, Surrey RH4 3YX
   Tel (0306) 881033

4. Tetra Fish Care
   Lambert Court
   Chestnut Avenue
   Eastleigh, Hants, SO5 3ZQ

These kits are simple, cheap and very useful. Errors may arise, however, due to lack of care in measuring the volumes of water and reagents. As well as this, any test based on a visual comparison of colour change is somewhat subjective and is open to differences in interpretation. For these reasons it may be preferrable for the Veterinarian to retest samples rather than to rely entirely on the client's own findings.

More accurate electronic meters are available to measure pH and Hardness. These, however, are relatively expensive.

The level of unionised ammonia cannot be measured directly, but is calculated from the TAN by taking account of the pH and temperature (See Chapter 2).

Salinity is very complex to measure by direct methods, and in practise it is calculated from a knowledge of the specific gravity using standard tables (See Appendix Six). Simple hygrometers are available to measure the specific gravity of water.

There are no simple or cheap test kits available to measure dissolved oxygen (D.O.) levels. Special meters are available from:

Barebo inc.
P.O. Box 217, B. D. 2,
Emmans, P. A. 18049
U.S.A.

These are probably too expensive for the general small animal practitioner.

Examination of the aquarium/pond system

If the water quality parameters are all within acceptable limits, there is unlikely to be a fault in the system. However, raised values would indicate that an examination of the system was necessary. Simple problems, such as incorrectly packed filter material, or kinked water pipes, may obviously prevent otherwise adequate equipment functioning correctly. A familiarity with the variety of equipment used in association with fishkeeping is essential (see chapters 3 & 4). The presence of dead animals, such as hedgehogs, frogs and birds may not have been noticed in the pond/filter system, but would obviously add to the level of toxic waste products in the water.

Examination of the system may fail to explain the presence of poor water quality. A careful history, however, might highlight a recent event that triggered the problem, and yet had itself since been rectified. In such a case, partial water changes may be all that are necessary until the system has re-equilibrated.

Consideration of the nitrogen cycle (chapter 2) would indicate that any event producing an imbalance of the filtration system would result in an initial peak in the ammonia level, followed by a subsequent peak in nitrite levels before equilibration is again established. Comparison of both the ammonia and nitrite levels is therefore useful in not only assessing the extent of the problem, but also the timescale involved:

A high ammonia with a low nitrite level would indicate a recent (probably 1-2 weeks) problem.

A moderate ammonia and nitrite level would indicate a slightly less recent problem (probably 2-3 weeks).

A low ammonia and a high nitrite level would indicate that the problem had occured some time ago (probably >3-4 weeks)

CHAPTER EIGHTEEN

RESTRAINT, HANDLING AND ANAESTHESIA

Lydia A Brown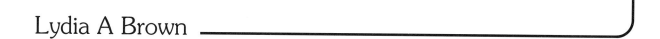

Anaesthetic agents are used for fish to reduce stress or pain. Although it is not clear the extent to which fish in fact feel pain, as a veterinarian, one should give these animals the benefit of the doubt. Fish ought to be tranquilised when handling them to avoid unnecessary trauma, which can result in scale damage and epidermal sloughing. It is possible to identify when a fish has been roughly held by observing the necrotic areas that develop some days later (usually around the wrist of the tail).

MANUAL RESTRAINT AND HANDLING

When manual restraint is a necessity, it is important to hold the fish firmly, yet gently. Since fish are extremely photophobic, their heads should be covered with a moist cloth if possible. Generally, the best method for grasping a large fish, is to hold it under the abdomen with one hand, using the fingers of that hand to hold onto the pectoral fins. The fingers should point in an anterior direction. The other hand firmly grasps the wrist of the tail.

Manual restraint may be used when the action to be taken on the fish is shorter than the time taken to anaesthetise the fish (for example transferring fish from one holding facility to another). Avoid excessive noise and jarring, and try to perform all movements smoothly.

It is possible to lower the basal metabolic rate of fish by lowering their body temperature. This can have the effect of making them easier to handle. However, this should be avoided wherever possible, since the act of lowering the water temperature can be a stressor. Nets which are used to transfer fish should be wide mouthed and made of material which is not likely to damage the scales of the fish.

ANAESTHESIA

Agents

There are a variety of anaesthetic agents which have been used in fish. A summary of the common ones, together with reported dose rates are given in Table 1.

In practice two agents are routinely used for fish. These are:

1. Tricaine methanesulphonate ("MS222") Sandoz Ltd. Basle, Switzerland

2. Ethyl-4-aminobenzoate ("Benzocaine") Non licensed, BDH Chemicals, Poole, Dorset.

Tricaine methanesulphonate and benzocaine are white crystalline compounds which are used at a particular concentration for anaesthesia, and at a lower concentration for tranquillisation. Tricaine methanesulphonate is soluble in water, and can be placed in the tank water directly. Benzocaine,

135

Table 1: Reported anaesthetic agents for fish

AGENT	SPECIES	COMMON NAME	DOSAGE
Chlorbutanol		Salmonids	2.8 – 3.5 mM/L
Ethanol in water	*F. parvipinnis*	Killifish	Anaesthesia not controllable
Ether	*C. auratus*	Goldfish	10 – 50 ml/L
Lidocaine	*T. mossambica*	Tilapia	Dosage very variable between species.
	C. carpio	Carp	Dosage very variable between species.
Lidocaine HCO_3			Better in adults than lidocaine. Use as combination of lidocaine (250 –350 mg/L) and $NaHCO_3$ (1 gm/L)
Methylparafynol	*F. parvipinnis*	Killifish	1.5 – 3.5 ml
Methylpentynol			0.5 – 0.9 ml/L
Pentobarbitone	*T. tinca*	Tench	2 mg/100 gm I/M
	R. rutilis	Roach	2 mg/100 gm I/M
2-Phenoxyethanol	*O. nerka*	Pacific salmon	0.1 – 0.5 ml/L
Procaine			0.25 – 1.0 ml, 5% solution intracranially
Propanidid	*C. carpio*	Carp	4 ml/L I/P
Propoxate	*C. auratus*	Goldfish	1 – 4 mg/L
Quinaldine sulphate		Tropical marines	200 mg/L
		Warm water spp.	15 – 70 mg/l
	R. pholis	Blenny	2.5 – 2 mg/L
Sodium amytal	*F. parvipinnis*	Killifish	Freshwater: 0.05 – 0.08 gm/L Saltwater: 0.4 – 0.65 gm/gal
Sodium bicarbonate	*C. carpio*	Carp	6.42 gm/L at pH 6.5
4-Styrylpyridine			20 – 50 mg/L
Tertiary-amyl alcohol	*F. parvipinnis*	Killifish	1 – 1.75 ml/L 0.5 – 1.1 ml/L
Etorphine/Acepromazine (Immobilon)	*C. auratus*	Goldfish	8 – 10 mg/kg (Recover with Revivon)

however, must first be dissolved in an organic solvent (usually ethanol, methanol or acetone). One major point to consider is that these compounds (especially tricaine methanesulphonate) are acidic, and a reduction of water pH can severely stress fish. If the local water supply is not well buffered, it may be necessary to use a phosphate or imidazole buffer to counter any decrease in pH.

Dose Rates

The doses generally recommended for use are:

1. Tricaine methanesulphonate (MS222)

   A 1:10,000 solution is considered an anaesthetic dose.
   A 1:20,000 solution is considered a tranquillising dose.
   A 1:30,000 solution or more dilute can be used for transportation of fish.

2. Benzocaine

   Either the same concentrations as for MS222 (as above) or: A stock solution of 100 grams of benzocaine in 1 litre of ethanol is prepared and stored in a dark glass container. This stock solution is added to the water containing the fish a few drops at a time until effects are noted.

When considering dosages, it is important to remember that each species of fish may react differently to anaesthesia, and **great care** should be taken. It is better to start with a very small dose, and work up to the standard dose with practice and experience.

Administration

Anaesthesia is administered topically, by placing the agent in water. There should always be an anaesthetic bath and a recovery bath with aeration provided, as well as the original container in which the fish was kept. If a large number of fish are to be anaesthetised, a small batch should first be anaesthetised and observed for signs of any delayed reaction, before proceeding with the whole batch.

Fish should ideally be starved for 12 to 24 hours before giving an anaesthetic agent. They may regurgitate if they have been offered food prior to anaesthesia, and in a small container, this reflux may give rise to clogging of the gills and cause trauma and/or asphyxiation. All containers should be at the same water temperature as that of the original one in which the fish arrived.

Signs of anaesthesia

These vary from species to species, but generally loss of balance occurs, followed by the fish rolling over so that the abdomen is uppermost. Initially, the fish cannot maintain its normal position. The fish may place its head in a corner of the tank. This is followed by a rolling motion, and finally the fish turns upside down. The fish may either stay on the bottom, or float to the surface. At first, gill movements are rapid, but as the fish becomes anaesthetised, these slow down. Handling the fish at this stage should provoke no reflex activity. If it does, the fish should be placed back in the anesthetic container until this reflex activity stops.

Fish may be taken out of the water, placed on a tray containing a moist paper towel, and procedures can be performed on the fish in this manner. The fish can be left in air for up to 5 minutes before it is placed in the recovery tank. If a longer procedure is anticipated, then the fish can be maintained on an anaesthetic solution using a recirculation system (See Brown [1987]). Good anaesthesia takes about 60-90 seconds to induce, and a similar time should be expected for full recovery. Induction should be smooth and relatively slow. In this manner it is possible to observe the fish through all the stages of anaesthesia as summarised in Table 2.

Recovery

This should take about 60-90 seconds and should not present a problem. However, if the fish fails to recover when placed in the recovery tank, it can be gently pushed in an antero-posterior direction so that freshwater passes over its gills. It is important never to allow water to flow past the gills of the fish in the opposite direction since this will cause irreparable damage to the gills.

In an emergency situation, the fish's head can be placed under a *gently* running coldwater tap for a minute, and then returned to the recovery tank. This has the action of flushing the anaesthetic solution over and away from the fish's gills. However, in areas of high chlorination, or fluorination, this is not recommended. Even after the gills have ceased to move, the heart of the fish beats for a long time, and so resuscitation should be attempted for a much longer period than would be expected for a warm blooded animal.

Table 2: Stages of Anaesthesia in Fish

STAGE	PLANE	DESCRIPTION SIGNS
1	1 Sedation	Reacts to stimuli: movement reduced
1	2 Sedation	Reduced reactivity to external stimuli; slight decrease in ventilation.
2	1 Light anaesthesia	Partial loss of equilibrium; fish rolls and attempts to right itself.
2	2 Deeper anaesthesia	Total loss of equilibrium; ventilation reduced.
3	Surgical anaesthesia	Failure to respond to any external stimuli: ventilation rate slow.
4	Medullary	No ventilation: cardiac arrest; collapse death.

[Adapted from McFarland, W.N. (1960): *The use of anesthetics for the handling and the transport of fishes*. Calif Fish Game **46**: 407-431.]

TRANSPORT

Fish which are to be transported may be tranquilised in the transport container. This reduces the basal metabolic rate of the fish, which in turn helps to prevent the build up of ammoniacal wastes and reduces the oxygen requirements of the fish. The water temperature may be chilled to aid in the same process. These procedures should be adopted if the fish are to be transported over any great distance, or for a long time. If fish are to be brought to a surgery for a consultation, then tranquillisation may not be necessary.

The same principles apply as for anaesthesia, although the fish must not lose its ability to maintain its normal swimming position. It is regrettable that all too frequently in commercial holdings, fish are transported at very high stocking densities. This is, of course, to be avoided. Polystyrene containers, or 'cool boxes', are ideal for carrying small numbers of fish. The fish should be placed in plastic bags in which aeration has been provided so as to supersaturate the water, or where battery operated air pumps can provide constant aeration.

EUTHANASIA

Euthanasia of fish should be taken seriously by the veterinarian and all practice staff, since clients develop as strong an attachment to their aquatic pets as to warm blooded animals. Small fish may be over-anaesthetised using a x 10 dose of the anaesthetic agent. When all movement has stopped, they can be finally euthanased by severing the spinal cord behind the gill covers. Larger fish can be dealt with in the same way, although with very large fish it may be impractical to do this. In such a case, a sharp blow to the head of the fish using a blunt wooden implement is given. Although this may be upsetting to observe, it is probably the kindest and quickest method for the fish.

CHAPTER NINETEEN

CLINICAL EXAMINATION OF FISH

Peter W Scott

This chapter assumes that a full clinical history and examination of the environment has already been carried out (Chapters 17 and 18). Such a strict separation of the clinical investigative approach is somewhat artificial due to the interdependancy of the subject, and the examination of the fish may prompt further investigations into the husbandry etc.

PRELIMINARY EXAMINATION OF THE FISH IN WATER

Fish should be viewed in the water (from above and from the side if possible), assessing their movements and respiratory rate. In general, fish movements are fluid and seeming relatively effortless. The respiratory movements are generally slow and not obvious. 'Wooden' movements, or marked respiratory movements should be viewed with suspicion.

Abnormal swimming movements and posture may be seen in fish with spinal deformities, generalised weakness, or CNS damage. Difficulty in maintaining normal body position in the water may result from any problems affecting the normal filling and emptying of the swimbladder, or from space occupying lesions etc. which may distort the swimbladder.

Abnormal movements will often be seen in response to skin irritation, such as that caused by ectoparasites. 'Flashing' involves sudden darting movements during which the fish flicks at the pond or tank bottom, rocks etc, exposing the lighter underside of the body, hence a 'flash' is seen. This needs to be distinguished from the normal feeding behaviour of many cyprinids, including koi. Fish may also jump due to irritation and this is often seen when they are parasitised with larger parasites such as *Argulus* spp. A certain amount of jumping is normal in koi, therefore treatment/quarantine tanks should always be covered.

Other abnormal movements seen in aquarium fish include 'shimmying'. This is a swimming-on-the-spot movement shown especially by livebearers (particularly black mollies, *Poecilia sphenops*) suffering from Myxobacterial skin infections. Certain species such as tiger barbs (*Barbus tetrazona*) show a 'headstanding-with-fins-erect' behaviour when suffering from nitrite toxicity, but this needs to be differentiated from similar behaviour shown by them when feeding. Individual fish species may show very bizarre swimming patterns such as headstanders (eg *Chilodus puncatus*), upside down catfish (*Synodontis nigriventris*) etc. Reference to textbooks such as Van Ramshorst (1978), or Mills et al (1988), may help to identify normal behaviour.

The behaviour of the fish in relation to others in its normal habitat (ie the pond or aquarium) can be informative. Many fish are social with their own or related species, and are normally seen in loose groups which form and reform, cruising the pond or aquarium. Fish which remain solitary or swim in a lethargic fashion away from the others may be unwell.

The position which fish adopt in relation to sources of oxygenated water can be highly significant. Fish with compromised oxygen transfer (gill conditions or anaemia) will seek out areas where oxygen levels are comparitively high. They may be seen 'mouthing' at the surface film of water, or close to the outlets of pumps, venturis, waterfalls or air stones. In heavily planted tanks or ponds diurnal fluctuations in oxygen levels may lead to this behaviour only being seen in the morning prior to the production of extra oxygen by photosynthesis. A curious sign described as 'coughing' involves a jerky movement with flared opercula. This is sometimes seen when gills are coated with mucus or irritated by suspended solids.

Fin carriage is also indicative of condition in the majority of fish and 'clamping' usually indicates that a fish is unwell.

DETAILED EXAMINATION OF THE FISH

Many of the following observations may be made with the fish in water, although they may require the fish to be confined in a plastic bag so that it can be examined from all angles. In general it is always worthwhile examining a fish this way if practicable since colour variations are much more difficult to assess with the fish out of water.

Skin

The skin in general should be smooth and unbroken and haemorrhages may suggest localised scale damage or more serious septicaemic problems. Fish skin differs from that of mammals because the whole epidermis is composed of living cells. This is then covered in a layer of mucus. When it is intact the skin and mucus layer of fish provide a waterproof coating (see chapter 1). The scales are embedded within the epidermis, and hence when scale loss occurs a serious skin defect is produced.

The scales should normally lay flat against the body. Lifting of scales to produce a 'pine-cone' effect may be due to localised or generalised anasarca associated often with abdominal swelling due to ascites. Localised intradermal or intra-abdominal lesions may produce smaller areas of lifted scales.

It may be possible to see larger ectoparasites such as leeches (eg *Piscicola* spp), anchor worm (*Lernaea* spp) or fish lice (*Argulus* spp). Certain of the smaller organisms may produce grossly recognisable signs on the skin surface. *Oodinium* spp may be seen as a fine golden dust, better seen with incident light, and this very fine appearance gives rise to the name Velvet Disease. White spots found anywhere on the body surface may be evidence of *Ichthyophthirius multifiliis* infection. In cyprinids such as goldfish, koi etc., these spots need to be differentiated from the sexual tubercles found all over the head, opercula and leading edges of the fins. Colour changes may also occur naturally as a response to changes in the environment or sex cycles etc (see chapter 1)

Black patches are seen with melanomas, especially in livebearers, and wild caught tropical fish or farmed coldwater fish may have obvious black spots within the skin caused by *Neascus* larvae.

Patches of apparent fungus may be true fungal infection, often due to *Saprolegnia* spp. These often have secondary green algal growth on them. A less 'fluffy' and much finer appearance is seen with myxobacterial infection (eg. mouth fungus in livebearers), and with *Epistylis* spp colonisation.

Identification of smaller parasites requires microscopic examination, but their presence may be suspected by behavioural changes, torn ragged fins or the presence of excess mucus. Excess mucus may be very obvious and hang in strands or may simply dull the fishes colours either over the whole fish or in patches. Changes in colour may also be seen with more generalised debilitating diseases such as Neon Tetra Disease or Fish tuberculosis. When handling fish a dry 'sand-paper' feel may result from long standing ectoparasitic infection through 'exhaustion' of the mucus-producing cells in the skin, this being particularly common with *Trichodina* spp infection.

Petechiation or larger haemorrhages may indicate a localised lesion, or may reflect a more generalised septicaemia/toxaemia. There may simply be erosion of the skin with consequent dermal damage (as mentioned above due to scale loss), fin rot lesions etc. In fish which have become severely affected and progressed to a septicaemia there may be hyperaemic skin wheals overlying muscle necrosis which may or may not progress to ulcers.

Fins may show lesions similar to those on the rest of the skin, and often begin to look raggy and frayed. Bacterial lesions are known to become chronic on the fins where the blood supply and immune response may be reduced. These often act as a source of infection when fish are later stressed.

Distinct nodules may be present on the skin, and these may be of varied consistancy. Jelly-like, haemorrhagic 'lumps' protruding between scales may be seen with *Dermocystidium koi* infection. Tumours can be seen, some of which may be associated with a variety of epithelial viral infections.

Lesions which look and feel similar to drops of candlewax found especially around the head and upper body are seen in koi carp suffering with carp pox. Lymphocystis, usually in marine fish, is associated with more roughened and cauliflower-like lesions. Granulomata may slowly erode, giving a different appearance to a 'normal' ulcer, generally showing a raised rim around a central crater. Detailed descriptions of such lesions are likely to be invaluable in making a diagnosis and prognosis for others.

Gills

During the overall assessment of the condition of the fish, it may be possible to catch a quick glimpse of the gills. In the majority of cases, however, it will be necessary to lightly anaesthetise the fish to examine the gills in detail. The gill can be seen by gently lifting the operculum and perhaps using a suitable light source to illuminate the buccal cavity. The gills should normally be a healthy 'salmon pink' colour, with clearly demarcated primary lamellae.

Many lesions may be seen including small white spots due to 'Ich'. Larger (1-2mm diameter) white cysts produced by myxosporideans may occur. Excess mucus may be present, coating sections or the whole gill surface. Sometimes a large erosion will be seen, due to the presence of *Dactylogyrus* spp or myxobacteria.

General palor may reflect anaemia, whereas haemorrhages may occur as a result of generalised septicaemia, viraemia, toxaemia or insults with chemicals or suspended solids.

Eyes

Eyes may show similar lesions to the skin. They should be checked for clarity of the cornea, opacities in the lens and haemorrhages in the adnexa. The eyes should also be examined for any signs of unilateral or bilateral exophthalmos. Bulging eyes or raised scales as seen in "Popeye" and "Dropsy" are the usual sequel to chronic bacterial lesions causing abdominal and retrobulbar effusion.

Internal organs

General observations may give some clue to gastro-intestinal function. Nematodes (*Camellanus* sp.) may be seen as a "red paintbrush" appearance protruding from the vent of some tropical fish. Trailing faeces may indicate constipation whereas translucent faeces may be associated with excess mucus production as seen with gastro-intestinal parasitism. More extensive examination of the viscera is possible, though this is uncommon.

Fish may be radiographed with or without the use of contrast media. The giving of barium using a stomach/oesophageal tube is relatively simple in anaesthetised fish. The use of rare earth screens etc is likely to be necessary to obtain the definition required.

Use of the laparoscope for examination of the proximal and distal portions of the alimentary tract is possible. The former route can be used in fish where the clinical history suggests an inability to eat, rather than an unwillingness. Abdominal laparoscopy is a straightforward technique with applications in fish, particularly for the biopsy of internal organs. In species such as koi however, the extremely adherent internal organ layout is likely to create difficulties.

Spinal abnormalities resulting from a range of causes from lightning strike to nutritional disorders have been investigated using this technique (Scott, unpublished data). Ultrasound, computerised tomography (CT Scanning) and magnetic resonance imaging (NMR) have all been applied to sharks (Stoskopf ,1990).

Further tests

Fish can be lightly anaesthetised and scrapings taken from skin and gills and examined for parasites. Blood can be taken ventrally from the caudal vein, although there may be difficulties in interpretation since the haematological parameters for a wide range of fish species are not known. Samples of faeces can be collected and examined for the presence of protozoa, nematode eggs etc. These are discussed more fully in chapter 20.

AUTOPSY PROCEDURES AND LABORATORY TECHNIQUES

Peter J Southgate
Edward J Branson

GENERAL CONSIDERATIONS

It is unfortunate that many of the symptoms exhibited by fish are common to a variety of diseases. The common signs of ill health (inappetence, lethargy, colour changes, fin-clamping and swelling of the abdomen and eyes) can all be caused by a number of aetiological agents. Although some specific symptoms, such as obvious irritation and flashing, or respiratory distress, may be suggestive of certain diseases, in most cases a more conclusive diagnosis will necessitate a certain amount of laboratory analysis.

The extent of laboratory analysis will frequently depend upon the problem under investigation, and the value of the fish to the client. In a population of numerous, relatively inexpensive fish, it is quite appropriate to sacrifice a few affected individuals in order to carry out a thorough clinical examination. This would not be possible when the problem concerns a small number of valued individuals. In the latter case, examination will be limited to a gross appearance and screening of fresh gill and skin preparations.

For a conclusive post mortem to be carried out, it is imperative that only very fresh material is examined. This is particularly true when histopathology is required, since fish tissue degenerates so quickly that taking samples even one hour after death could give results which are of little diagnostic use.

Ideally living, but obviously affected or moribund fish should be sacrificed for examination. Failing that, samples should be taken from a fish as soon after death as possible. Those taken from frozen fish are invariably useless.

EXAMINATION OF FRESH GILL SQUASHES

Introduction

Gill squashes are useful in determining the presence of parasites, and may be of use in the assessment of general gill health and local bacterial and fungal infections.

Ensure that the water in which the fish is kept prior to examination is well oxygenated to maintain the viability of any parasites present.

Technique - sampling from a recently sacrificed fish

A gill squash is prepared as follows:

1. Using scissors or a scalpel blade, remove a small number of primary lamellae from the gill arch (do not include any cartilage). It is often advisable not to use the outermost arch, which is sometimes in poor condition, and may give a false impression of the general health of the gill.

2. Place the gill tissue on a microscope slide, add a small amount of water. Apply a cover slip with sufficient pressure to allow the filaments to spread and fan out. Always prepare a gill squash using the water in which the fish were submitted. Avoid tapwater or distilled water, as the presence of chlorine, or a change in osmotic pressure, may destroy any parasites present. Examine immediately.

3. The majority of protozoan and metazoan parasites can be visualised using a microscope with a 40X magnification (i.e: a 10X eyepiece and a 4X objective). Some of the smaller protozoa are more difficult to see, and may need a 10X objective. It is never necessary to use a higher magnification for the detection of parasites.

Technique - sampling from live fish

In a fish that is not to be sacrificed for clinical examination, it is not be possible to remove gill tissue, but an impression smear can be obtained from an anaesthetised fish without harm, by pressing a dry microscope slide against the gill tissue. It may be possible to do this in an unanaesthetised specimen held gently in a wet towel. If possible, the latter method is preferable, as there is a possibility that the anaesthetic agent may affect any parasites present.

Mucus and parasites from the gill will adhere to the slide and, with the addition of a small amount of water and a cover slip, can be examined microscopically. If concerned about harming the gill tissue using this technique in valuable fish, it is possible to get an idea of the presence of gill parasites by taking a sample of mucus from the skin adjacent to the gill.

The provision of phase contrast on a microscope often assists the detection of parasites, but if this is not available, lowering the condenser to increase the depth of field of the image often helps to make the parasites more visible.

Interpretation

Gill squashes can have some use in assessing the general condition of the gill tissue. The gill epithelium can react to an insult in a very limited number of ways. It can produce a lot of mucus in an attempt to protect itself against damage, and to 'wash away' irritating particles or parasites. If the insult persists, the epithelial cells can proliferate (hyperplastic response) in a further attempt to protect itself from damage.

Both these reactions may, with sufficient experience, be seen when examining a gill squash. Epithelial proliferation appears as an apparent thickening and 'clubbing' of the ends of the gill filaments, or fusion of adjacent areas of the gill. However, the assessment of gill health by means of fresh gill squashes must be considered with caution, as it relies heavily on the technique and experience of the operator. The appearance of a gill in a fresh preparation may often be contradicted by its histological appearance.

The presence of myxobacteria can also be determined in fresh gill preparations. These will frequently be found in cases of environmental gill disease, and often accompany increased levels of mucus and particulate matter. Myxobacteria can be present in such large numbers that grossly they have a 'cotton wool' appearance on the gill. Individual bacteria can be readily seen in fresh gill preparations, but it is usually necessary to use a higher magnification than that used for parasite screening (i.e: a 40X objective). They appear as filamentous rods, usually motile (described as a gliding motion), and often clumping together (see chapter 11).

Fungal infection (principally *Saprolegnia*), may also be identified in gill squashes. Hyphae are much larger than the myxobacteria, and can be easily seen with a 10X objective.

EXAMINATION OF FRESH SKIN SCRAPES

Skin scrapes are useful in the same way as gill squashes, to detect the presence of ectoparasites, bacteria and fungi on the skin.

Technique

Skin scrapes are prepared in much the same way as gill squashes:

1. Using a scalpel blade or the end of a slide, a small quantity of mucus is removed from the skin. As parasites often concentrate in the areas adjacent to, and protected by, the fins it is useful to take the scrapings from these areas.

2. Apply a drop of water and a cover slip and examine using exactly the same technique as that described for gill squashes.

Skin scrapes, like gill squashes, are used principally for the detection of ectoparasites, but may also reveal the presence of fungi or myxobacterial infection.

If the fish under examination is to be sacrificed, a complete post mortem can be carried out. Fish are usually sacrificed by rapidly severing the spinal cord just behind the gill covers with a sharp blade, or by means of a sharp blow to the head (chapter 18). Anaesthetic overdose is an appropriate alternative, but some ectoparasites could be removed using this technique.

POST-MORTEM EXAMINATION

As stressed above, it is very important that a post mortem is carried out while the fish is very fresh, and samples for histological examination are obtained as soon after death as possible.

Equipment required

The equipment needed to carry out a post mortem is very basic:

> Dissection board
> Dissection kit
> Microscope, slides, cover slips
> Fixative in leak-proof pots for histological samples

In addition, if bacteriological sampling is to be carried out:

> Bunsen and gas source
> Bacteriological loop, disposable sterile loops, or swabs
> Agar plates - specialised media
> Incubator

Technique

Technique will vary with the problem under investigation and the extent of analysis carried out, but the following describes the majority of procedures necessary for a thorough clinical examination.

1. Examine the fish for the presence of gross external abnormalities. Factors to consider include:

   a) Skin: Variation in colour
   Excess mucus production
   Gross lesions (e.g: ulcers, haemorrhages, scale loss)
   Parasites visible to the naked eye (e.g: *Argulus*)
   Apparent fungal infection
   Tumours

   b) Fins: Loss of fin or tail
   Fin or tail erosions ('rot')
   Haemorrhages, particularly at the base of the fin
   Apparent fungal infection
   Tumours

c) Eye: Evidence of damage
Corneal opacity or ulceration
Cataract
Tumours
d) Other gross abnormalities
(e.g: opercular damage, abdominal swelling, protruding haemorrhagic vent, spinal deformity).

2. Obtain fresh gill and skin preparations as detailed above (FIGS. 1 & 2).

FIG. 1 : Skin Scraping and exposure of gills.

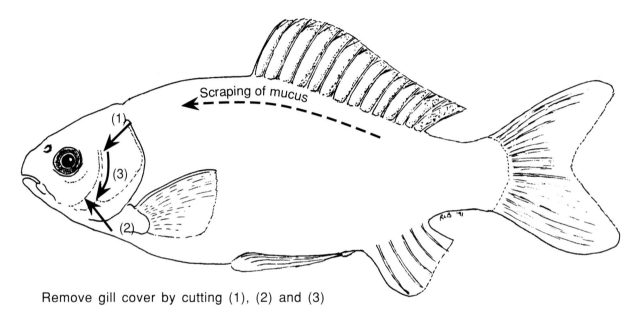

Remove gill cover by cutting (1), (2) and (3)

FIG 2 : Sampling of gill arch.

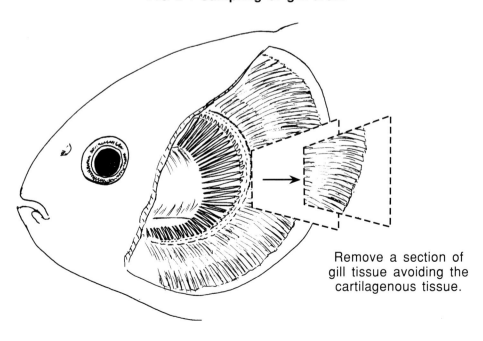

Remove a section of gill tissue avoiding the cartilagenous tissue.

3.   Carry out an internal examination. The following applies mostly to fish large enough to examine (the post-mortem examination of very small fish may be limited). As discussed in chapter 1, the presence, appearance and distribution of the abdominal organs is very variable in different species, and the accompanying description and diagrams relate to carp.

The technique involves the following stages:

1.   The abdomen of the fish is opened by cutting along the ventral midline, from the opercular region to the vent. Avoid opening the gut and spilling the intestinal contents (this is especially important if bacteriological examination is to be carried out). (FIG.3)

     Improved exposure of the abdominal viscera may be achieved by making a second cut extending in an antero-dorsal direction from the distal end of the primary incision. The whole lateral abdominal wall can then be reflected forwards and removed. (FIGS. 3 & 4)

2.   The abdominal organs can be visualised more easily by gently using a seeker or forceps to separate them. The gonads can be reflected caudally (FIG. 5), and the bowel loops ventrally (FIG. 6), to expose the swimbladder and a portion of the kidney.

3.   Note the presence of any gross abnormality of the abdominal contents - haemorrhage, parasite cysts, tumours, swim-bladder abnormalities etc.
     Note the consistency and colour of the liver.
     Note the presence and nature of any free abdominal fluid.

4.   If bacteriological examination is to be carried out, it should be performed at this stage (see below). This will require adequate exposure of the kidney, which can be achieved by grasping the caudal pole of the swimbladder with forceps, and reflecting it cranially (FIG. 7).

5.   The stomach and gut are opened, and the contents examined for evidence of feeding. The nature of the gut contents and the presence of gut parasites are noted. Large metazoan parasites, such as tapeworms etc., can be removed for later identification (preserved in 5% formalin if necessary) and a gut scrape can be prepared in exactly the same manner as that used for skin scrapes, for the detection of protozoa, such as *Hexamita* sp.

6.   Samples should now be taken for histopathological examination.

FIG 3: Opening the abdominal cavity

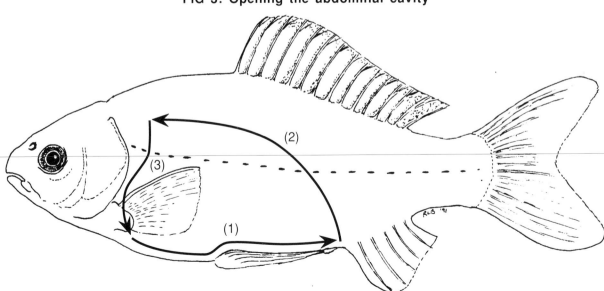

Incise along lines (1), (2)and (3) and reflect
off lateral body wall.

FIG.4 : Exposed abdominal viscera *in situ*.

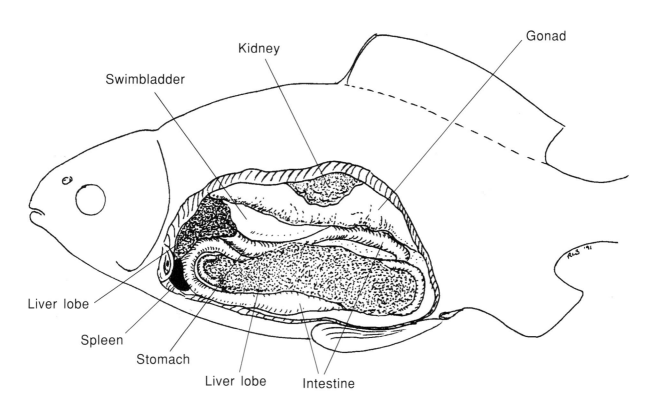

FIG 5 : Caudal reflection of the gonads.

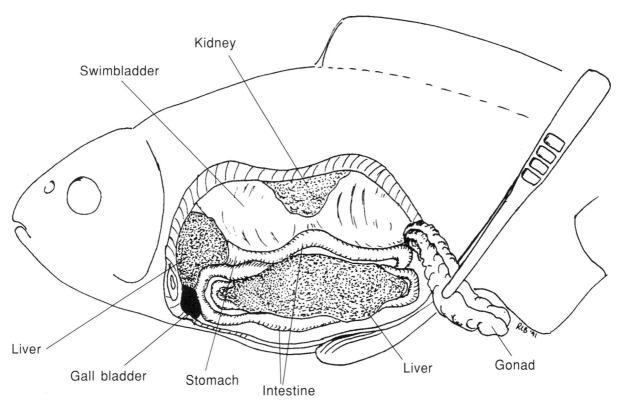

FIG 6 : Ventral reflection of the bowel.

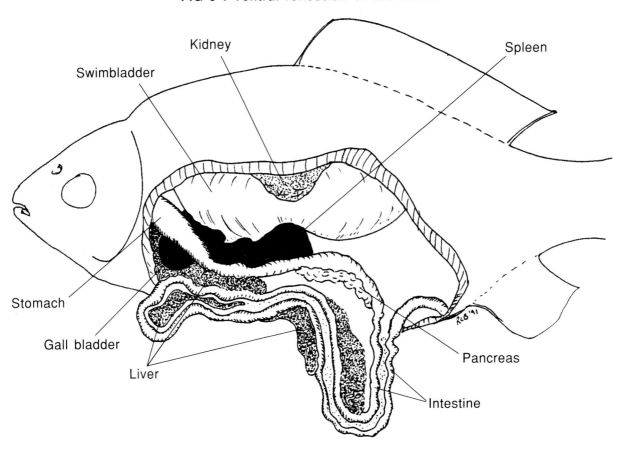

FIG 7 : Exposure of the kidney

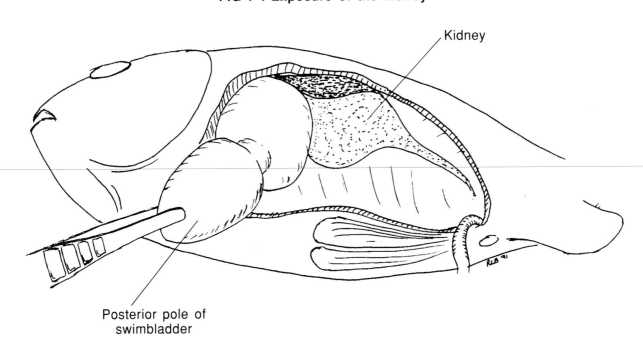

HISTOPATHOLOGY

Sampling tissue

Pieces of tissue no larger than one cubic centimetre are taken from the following organs:

i.   Gill - cut out a section of gill arch approx. $^1/_2$ cm wide. It is preferable to take the sample from the second gill arch, as the outer one is prone to damage, and may give an unrepresentative histological appearance.

ii. Skin/muscle - a block of skin/muscle removed across the lateral line gives a good representation of red and white muscle and also includes the fat body around the lateral line.

iii. Spleen

iv. Intestine - pyloric caecae and fat which will include the pancreas when present.

v.   Liver

vi. Kidney

vii. Heart

The above organs are those most usually screened during histopathological examination, but if any gross abnormalities are noted in other tissues (e.g: eye, swimbladder, fin etc.), these should also be included for analysis.

If a relatively small fish is submitted for examination, then it is not usually possible to sample individual organs for histopathology. As a rule of thumb, a fish with a body depth of less than 1cm (assuming a standard fish shape) would not be sampled in the above manner, but the body can be cut into $^1/_2$ cm 'steaks' (transverse sections from the head to the tail) and all sections fixed. An alternative to this would be to open the abdomen, tease out the abdominal contents and fix the whole fish. There is a danger, however, that in all but the very smallest fish, this latter procedure will not give adequate fixation of the tissues.

Fixatives

The standard fixative for fish histology is 10% neutral buffered formalin (formula at the end of the chapter). Other fixatives, such as formol saline and Bouin's fluid can also be used.

It is important that a sufficient volume of fixative is used to ensure adequate fixation of the tissues - at least 20X volume of formalin to tissue. For ease of posting, it is acceptable to fix tissue in a large volume of formalin for 24 hours and then greatly reduce the volume of fixative before forwarding to the laboratory.

Postage to the laboratory

Standard guidelines for posting pathological specimens should be followed (obtainable from the Post-Office or RCVS) and it is advisable to contact the laboratory to inform them of the material being submitted, and possibly to discuss details of the case under examination.

In general, the tissue samples should be sealed in leak-proof containers, suitably labelled. These should be packed in absorbent material, in a rigid container or padded bag, enclosing a detailed history. The package should be labelled 'pathological specimen - with care' and sent by first class post to the diagnostic laboratory.

BACTERIOLOGY

General considerations

The extent of bacteriological analysis that can be carried out will depend on the facilities available, and the expertise of the operator. In the majority of cases, the limit of examination will be obtaining a primary inoculum on appropriate media which is then forwarded to the diagnostic laboratory. Some practices will be equipped to carry out basic bacteriological identification - gram staining, motility tests etc (see below), but more sophisticated techniques, such as biochemical tests, serology etc., are outside the scope of this manual, and the reader is directed to more specialised texts.

Sampling

External lesions can be examined for the presence of bacteria by searing the lesion with a hot scalpel blade and inserting a sterile bacteriological loop. The inoculum on the loop can then be plated out using standard technique (see later).

It must be emphasised that, because of the intimate contact of the fish with its aquatic environment, and the many bacterial species commonly present in the water, contamination of bacterial plates with naturally-occurring aquatic organisms will often occur with samples taken from skin/fin lesions and may give misleading results. These results must be interpreted very carefully to gauge the significance of the isolated bacteria.

The kidney is the organ most frequently sampled for bacteriological analysis. It is usually a simple procedure to obtain an uncontaminated inoculum and, because of it's importance as a blood-forming organ, as well as an organ of excretion, it's extensive vascular supply ensures that any organism causing a bacteraemia or septicaemia is likely to be found in samples from this tissue.

A sample is obtained after having cleanly removed the swimbladder and exposing the surface of the kidney. In most fish this capsule is easily penetrated using the bacteriological loop, but in larger fish, where the kidney capsule is tough, this may need incising with a sterile scalpel before the sample is taken.

Direct examination of Gram stained kidney smears may also give an indication of the presence of bacteria. This is performed by emulsifying a small portion of kidney in distilled water on a slide, air drying, and then heat fixing the material. The slide is then stained using the Gram technique, and examined at 400X or 1000X magnification. Similarly prepared slides may be stained with Ziehl-Neelsen stain and examined for the presence of acid-fast bacilli.

Direct inoculation of agar plates

The sample is taken by inserting a sterile loop (either wire or disposable plastic) into the body of the kidney and obtaining a sufficient amount of kidney tissue to inoculate an agar plate. Ensure that the area of kidney used for the sample is not that which is to be used for histopathological analysis.

In small fish, it is difficult to take useful bacteriological samples, although it may be possible to cut through the body exposing the cut surface of the kidney which could then be seared with a hot scalpel, and a bacteriological sample taken by inserting a sterile wire into the kidney tissue.

The inoculum on the loop is 'plated out' onto the agar by using the standard bacteriological technique of spreading the material onto a segment of the plate and then, using a re-sterilized or new plastic loop, streaking the sample onto a second segment of the plate. This procedure is continued until the whole plate is utilised (FIG.8). This technique ensures that the material on the loop is diluted out over the plate, and aids the isolation of single bacterial colonies for identification.

FIG.8 : Plating out an inoculum onto agar

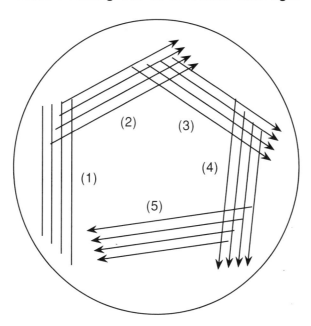

Bacteriological culture

Many of the bacterial fish pathogens described in this manual can be successfully cultured on standard bacteriological media, tryptone soya agar (TSA) being the most frequently used (see formula at end of chapter). Some of the pathogens are difficult to culture, however, needing specialised media and culture conditions. This is the case with the Myxobacteria (where the diagnosis is usually based on the examination of fresh gill and skin preparations and histological examination of tissues), and *Mycobacterium* sp. (where histological examination is usually required for the diagnosis). If these conditions are suspected, an attempt can be made to culture the bacteria on specialised media, but results from this are frequently disappointing, and it is advisable to rely on the other diagnostic techniques to identify the presence of these organisms.

If bacterial disease is suspected in marine fish, sampling onto a marine agar, or TSA with added salt, in addition to standard TSA, will facilitate the isolation of organisms such as *Vibrio* sp.

Sterile disposable swabs can be used for bacteriological sampling of fish, but it is necessary to plate these out onto agar as soon as possible, as fish pathogens will not survive for long on the swab. Various transport media have been tried for fish bacteria, but nothing satisfactory has yet been found.

The sampled plates can then be forwarded to an appropriate laboratory, taking adequate precautions to protect the plates from damage. The use of a proprietary sealing film to seal the plates against the ingress of foreign material is recommended.

If facilities are available, a certain amount of bacteriological identification can be carried out at the practice. Inoculated plates must be incubated and examined every day for evidence of bacterial growth. The standard temperature for incubation of bacterial fish pathogens is 22°C, and most will grow well within seven days. Other temperatures may be needed with certain species (see chapter 11).

Bacteriological culture - difficulties in interpretation

If any growth is observed on the plates, it is important that any further examination or identification is carried out on bacterial colonies which are likely to be of significance in the disease under investigation. It is extremely easy to obtain a mixed growth of bacteria, which may include bacterial fish pathogens, but may also contain contaminants and aquatic organisms not involved in disease.

This is particularly true if culturing bacteria from external lesions. This emphasises the need for aseptic technique, and also for the 'diluting'effect of plating out material to obtain single colonies on the plate. If a mixed culture is obtained, sometimes one organism will predominate. This may appear, on the face of it, to be the most significant organism present, but this may not be the case. Until experienced in bacteriological examination, it will therefore be necessary to look at all the different colonies present.

Whether a pure growth of bacteria, or a mixed growth has been obtained, it is preferable to subculture individual colonies on to fresh plates and incubate these. This allows a check to be made on the purity of the subculture, and gives enough pure growth to carry out the various identification techniques. Of course it also takes longer to do this, and if rapid identification is needed, then this will need to be carried out on the primary culture. However, it is imperative that a pure growth of an apparently significant organism is used to do this. Much valuable time may be wasted in running tests on an insignificant bacterium, after having picked the wrong colony from a mixed culture on the primary plate.

Bacteriological examination - basic information required

Generally, it may not be necessary to establish the specific identity of the bacterium involved in the infection. It is only really necessary:

a)   To be sure that bacteria are playing a significant role in the disease under investigation (i.e: the problem is a true bacterial disease). This is only possible from experience of similar problems, from the clinical history and from having obtained a good pure growth of bacteria.

b)   If a treatment is indicated, to discover the antibiotic sensitivity of the organism.

BACTERIOLOGICAL IDENTIFICATION - FURTHER TESTS

A few of the basic tests that can be carried out are detailed below. Precise identification of organisms by means of biochemical and serological tests is not considered.

Gram stain

This is the standard stain used to show the general morphology of the bacteria, as well as categorising them by their Gram reaction. It is possible to carry out a Gram stain on smears of kidney material to visualise any bacteria present, and give an indication of bacterial septicaemia.

The technique involves the following steps:

1.   A small quantity of bacterial culture or kidney material is emulsified in distilled water on a clean slide.
2.   The slide is air dried and then heat fixed by passing it a few times through the bunsen flame.
3.   The cooled slide is placed on a staining rack and stainedfor one minute with crystal violet solution
4.   The crystal violet is washed off with iodine, and the slide stained with fresh iodine for one minute.
5.   The iodine is washed off with repeated flushes of alcohol/acetone until no more colour washes off the slide.
6.   The slide is washed with water.
7.   Excess water is shaken off and the slide stained with safranin for two minutes.
8.   The slide is washed with water and dried.
9.   Examine the stained slide under 400X magnification and then under oil immersion at 1000X magnification.

Gram positive bacteria appear blue/purple
Gram negative bacteria appear red/pink

The Gram staining technique is notoriously difficult to get absolutely correct, and practise is needed for consistent results to be obtained.

Ziehl-Neelsen Stain

This technique is used to demonstrate *Mycobacterium* sp. and other acid-fast organisms. It involves the following steps:

1. An air dried, heat fixed smear is prepared as above.
2. Apply prepared Carbol Fuchsin solution, and heat until steam rises. Keep the stain hot for 5 minutes, but do not boil or allow the stain to dry on the slide.
3. Wash with water.
4. Apply several changes of acid-alcohol solution until the preparation is colourless or faint pink.
5. Wash with water.
6. Apply methylene blue solution for 20 to 30 seconds.
7. Wash with water,blot carefully and dry with gentle heat.

Motility test

This test will differentiate between motile and non-motile organisms. Many bacteria are capable of motility by the presence of flagellae. Although motility can be determined by the direct observation of bacteria on a microscope slide (a small quantity of bacteria dispersed in a drop of sterile saline under a cover slip), it is preferable to use a technique where the organisms are observed suspended in a 'hanging drop'.

The 'hanging drop' technique involves the following steps:

1. Soft paraffin is used to support a cover slip above a microscope slide. This is achieved by placing a small quantity of the paraffin on the four corners of the cover slip.
2. Onto the centre of the cover slip, on the same side as the paraffin, is placed a loopful of sterile saline (remember to sterilise the loop first).
3. Using a sterile loop, a small quantity of bacteria from the culture is emulsified carefully in the saline.
4. A clean slide is then lowered onto the paraffin and the slide inverted so that the bacterial suspension is hanging as a drop from the cover slip above the microscope slide. The suspension must not touch the slide.
5. Examine this preparation under the microscope at 400X magnification, taking care not to touch the cover slip with the objective of the microscope.

Motile bacteria should be seen moving in a non-random, directional motion (i.e: non-Brownian motion).

FIG 9 : The hanging drop

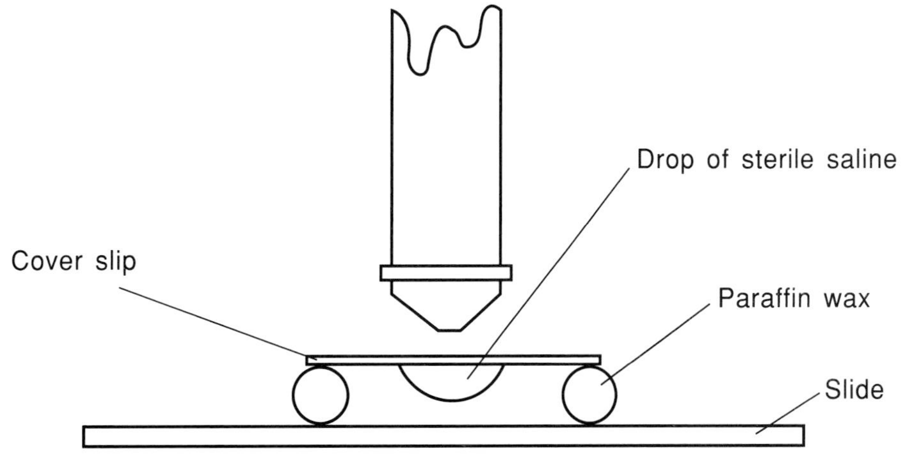

Oxidation/fermentation (O/F) test

This is useful in further differentiating bacteria, and demonstrates whether the organism breaks down glucose aerobically or anaerobically.

Screw-topped test tubes containing O/F medium and a sterile straight wire (not a loop) are required, and the technique involves the following steps:

1. Using the sterile wire, an inoculum of pure bacterial culture is stabbed into the O/F medium in one tube and the top replaced. Aseptic technique must be observed at all times.

2. A second tube is inoculated in exactly the same way, but a 1cm layer of liquid paraffin is placed on the surface of the medium to exclude any air before the top is replaced.

3. The two tubes are incubated, and any colour change in the medium is noted.

    The conclusions made from the results can be summarised as follows:

Aerobic tube	Anaerobic tube	Conclusion
Green	Green.	No reaction on glucose
Blue at top	Green	Alkaline reaction
Yellow	Yellow	Oxidative
Yellow	Yellow	Fermentative

Oxidase test

This is a further simple biochemical test which indicates whether the bacteria are in possession of certain oxidase enzymes. For this test a reagent strip (the oxidase strip) is required. A platinum wire is also needed. The technique involves:

1. Using a sterile platinum wire an inoculum of pure culture is smeared onto the area of the strip containing the oxidase reagent.

2. Note any colour change in the strip over the following minute.

A purple colour developing within a minute indicates a positive result.

ANTIBIOTIC SENSITIVITY TESTING

Antibiotic sensitivity testing is advisable in all cases of possible bacterial disease. This will help to indicate a suitable treatment and identify any antibiotic resistance being exhibited by the bacterium.

Antibiotic sensitivity discs of appropriate strength may be obtained from the pharmaceutical companies supplying compounds licensed for fish use.

As emphasised above, it is extremely important that, when carrying out antibiotic sensitivity testing, a pure culture of the primary pathogen is used. Totally misleading results will be obtained if the susceptibility of a non-important commensal or contaminant bacterium or a mixed culture is used for this test.

Technique

1. Remove several colonies of bacteria from pure growth on an agar plate using a sterile loop.

2. Inoculate the bacteria into a small volume of sterile distilled water in a sterile bijou (or similar) bottle. Do this by rubbing the bacteria onto the inside surface of the bottle rather than placing the loop in the water; try to avoid touching the neck of the bottle with the loop or the fingers. Replace the bottle cap.

3. Suspend the bacteria in the water by gentle shaking.

4. Using a sterile pipette, place a few drops of this suspension onto the surface of an agar plate. The agar used most frequently for this is sensitest agar (see end of chapter), although TSA can be used. Spread this suspension over the surface of the agar using a sterile loop or glass spreader. Allow the plate to dry for a minute or two.

5. Place antibiotic sensitivity discs on the surface of the agar, equidistant from each other and the edge of the plate.

6. Invert the plate and incubate at an appropriate temperature.

7. When a good growth of bacteria is visible on the plate, the antibiotic sensitivity of the organism is shown by the absence of bacterial growth around the sensitivity disc (the zone of inhibition). The size of this zone will reflect, to some extent, the degree of susceptibility of the bacterium to that antibiotic (the larger the zone, the more susceptible the bacterium), and the drug of choice is likely to be that exhibiting the largest zone of inhibition.
    It must be borne in mind that this test does not replicate the true clinical conditions of fish receiving antibiotic treatment, but does help in deciding the most effective treatment to use.

VIROLOGICAL SAMPLING

Analysis of fish tissues for the presence of virus infection can only be carried out by specialised laboratories and, if virus infection is suspected, it is preferable to contact a competent laboratory to discuss the most appropriate sampling procedure. Often it is possible to submit live fish for examination, although freshly-dead fish or tissue samples submitted on ice may be acceptable. It is advisable to get the tissues to the laboratory within 24 hours of sampling. Virological analysis can be very expensive.

BLOOD SAMPLING

Haematology is a very little explored field in ornamental fish. Very few blood parameters, for very few species have been ascertained, and although it is hoped that fish haematology will become a useful tool in the future, at present blood analysis is restricted to the examination of fresh blood smears for the presence of parasites. Blood samples can be taken by caudal venipuncture or direct from the heart using a hypodermic syringe or vacutainer. For a blood smear, however, it is perfectly acceptable to take a drop of blood from the heart, gill or other tissue during a post mortem. This is examined microscopically using standard technique.

TOXICOLOGY

The samples required, and the method of sampling is discussed fully in chapter 13.

FIXATIVES FOR FISH TISSUES

Phosphate-buffered Formalin

40% Formaldehyde	100ml
Tap/distilled water	900ml
Sodium dihydrogen phoshate ($NaH_2PO_4H_2O$)	4g
Disodium hydrogen phosphate (Na_2HPO_4)	6g

Bouin's Fluid

Saturated aqueous picric acid	75ml
Formalin	25ml
Acetic acid	5ml

CULTURE MEDIA FOR THE ISOLATION OF FISH PATHOGENIC BACTERIA

Tryptone Soya Agar (TSA) (Oxoid)

Tryptone	15.0	g/litre
Soya peptone	5.0	g/litre
Sodium chloride	5.0	g/litre
Agar No. 3	15.0	g/litre

Final pH : 7.3

Marine Agar

This is TSA with the final salt concentration adjusted to 2% to favour the growth of marine organisms.

Sensitest Agar

Hydrolysed casein	11.0	g/litre
Peptones	3.0	g/litre
Sodium chloride	3.0	g/litre
Dextrose	2.0	g/litre
Starch	1.0	g/litre
Buffer salts	3.3	g/litre
Nucleoside bases	0.02	g/litre
Thiamine	0.00002	g/litre
Agar No. 1	8.0	g/litre

Final pH : 7.4

CHAPTER TWENTY ONE

THERAPEUTICS

Peter W Scott

At the time of writing much of the legislation on the use of 'water' treatments is in flux. Certain compounds such as malachite green are likely to disappear, and most of the proprietary medicines will probably change radically or be removed from sale. This in turn may increase the numbers of aquarists calling on veterinary surgeons for help.

Depending on the type of disease and the individual situation, sick fish should be either removed and treated separately in isolation, or kept with the rest of the fish and all treated collectively. Outbreaks of contagious disease are best dealt with *en masse*, but fish affected with certain bacterial diseases should be treated individually. Fish affected with large visible parasites such as Anchor worm (*Lernaea* spp) and fish lice (*Argulus* spp) should be treated individually to remove adults but treated with the rest of the apparently healthy fish to remove the larvae.

ANTIBACTERIALS

Treatment via the water is always a very poor second to inclusion of a treatment antibiotic into the food of the fish. Hard water in particular tends to cause problems, since it chelates tetracyclines and renders them useless except in very high doses. When used at lower doses the microorganisms living in the aquarium are exposed to levels which tend to cause antibiotic resistance. The choice of antibiotics is often suggested initially by experience and then later modified by "sensitivity testing".

Antibacterials administered via the water

N.B. This route is of limited use and should not to be used in systems dependent on bacterial filtration. It may, however, be necessary to use this route when fish are not feeding by setting up a separate treatment tank where water quality can be controlled by regular water changes. Calcium levels in hard water areas will often interfere with certain antibiotics by chelating them and effectively reducing availability (Gratzek, 1981).

Table 1: Suggested doses of antibacterials administered via the water

Oxytetracycline	13-120mg/litre (chelated by hard water)
Doxycycline & Minocycline	2-3mg/litre
Chloramphenicol	20-50mg/litre
Potentiated sulphonamide	(80mg trimethoprim & 400mg sulphadiazine per ml) used at 1ml/100-120 litres
Nifurpirinol	0.1mg/litre
Metronidazole	7mg/litre (double for Oodinium)
Dimetridazole	5mg/litre (said to inhibit spawning)
Neomycin	50mg/kg (used in seawater)
Gentamycin	4-5mg/kg (used in seawater)
Kanamycin	50-100mg/litre
Nitrofurazone	1-3mg/litre

Antibacterials administered via the food

In the UK, four antibiotics are in relatively common usage among farmed fish. These are:

Oxytetracycline	Microtet: Microbiologicals, Pharmsure Tetraplex: PH Pharmaceuticals
Oxolinic acid	Pharmsure Aquinox: PH Pharmaceuticals Aqualinic Powder: Parke Davis
Potentiated sulphonamide	Tribrissen: Pitman-Moore Sulphatrim: PH Pharmaceuticals
Amoxycillin	Aquacil: PH Pharmaceuticals Vetremox: Vetrepharm

There are also currently available medicated flake foods, Aquaflake and Oxyflake (PH Pharmaceuticals) containing oxolinic acid and oxytetracycline respectively. Specialist manufacturers of flake foods (King British) may also make up large amounts on receipt of a VWD (Veterinary Written Direction).

A number of other antibiotics have been used with success in fish. **Erythromycin** compounds have been of value in certain aspects of the control of Bacterial Kidney Disease (BKD), and drugs such as **clindamycin** and **kitasamycin** also have shown promise (Stoker, personal communication). **Naladixic** acid (closely related to oxolinic acid) seemed in the laboratory to be potentially useful in treating enteric redmouth (ERM) but in practical use failed (Scott, unpublished data).

As a general rule fish will be medicated by mixing antibiotics onto food, although there are certain ready-medicated foods available on veterinary prescription.

The fish will be given approximately 0.25% of their body weight per day as medicated pelleted food. In fish farming, where greater amounts of food are used, a routine feed rate for medicated food is often 1% of body weight. Although feeding rates of up to 3-4% body weight are reported for tropical fish (Klontz, personal communication), observations of feed rates used in koi dealerships and home ponds show that these are more commonly in the region 0.25-0.5%.

Table 2: Quantities of drug added to fish feed

	PERCENTAGE BODY WEIGHT TO BE FED			
	0.25%	0.5%	1.0%	2.0%
1kg of food feeds for 1 day	400kg	200kg	100kg	50kg
OTC 50mg/kg fish pure	20g	10g	5g	2.5g
Furazolidone 75mg/kg fish pure	30g	15g	7.5g	3.75g
Potentiated sulphonamide 30mg/kg fish pure	12g	6g	3g	1.5g
40%	30g	15g	7.5g	3.75g
Oxolinic acid 10mg/kg fish pure	4g	2g	1g	0.5g
50%	8g	4g	2g	1g
Amoxycillin 80mg/kg fish pure	32g	16g	8g	4g

Oral Antibacterials in Marine fish

Care needs to be taken transposing dose rates from freshwater to seawater since there are major differences in the physiology of fish from these respective environments (O'Grady et al 1986). There seems to be a much reduced uptake of quinolones (oxolinic acid and flumequin), and a similar but not so marked reduction with oxytetracycline. Because of the increased concentration of urine in seawater, sulphonamides can be dangerous due to their potential for forming crystals in the urine (Wood and Johnson, 1957).

Dosages are often modified as follows:

Oxolinic acid	30mg/kg	
Oxytetracycline	75mg/kg	
Tribrissen	30-50mg/kg	(double dose on day 1)

This area is one fraught with traps for the unwary, and great caution should be exercised. Excessively high levels of antibiotics are thought to be even more likely to cause resistance than low levels and this may be a factor in the rapid development of resistance to the quinolones in seawater farms.

The use of oxytetracycline at low levels has been linked with immunosuppression in carp. Rijkers, 1980 suggested that the humoral immune response might be susceptible to low levels of oxytetracycline, although the cellular response remained unaffected.

Practical home medication

A useful recipe for producing a home-medicated feed (using metronidazole as an example) is: 250g ox heart + 7g wheat germ + 7g chopped spinach, liquidise and add 15 x 200 mg metronidazole, solidify using 75ml of 10% gelatin

Alternative foods can be made by simply pulverising flake food and adding a flavouring agent such as spinach or prawns as appropriate. Vitamin products such as ACE-High (Vetark), and antibiotics can then be added. The whole mix can then be 'set' using gelatin or agar. Ice cube trays can be used to hold such foods so that a block can be popped out easily.

Antibacterials by injection

This is a preferred route of administration when fish are of a suitable size. It is of particular value when initiating treatment which may then be continued by the oral route. Suitable drugs and dosages include:

Ampicillin	10mg/kg daily
Chloramphenicol succinate	40mg/kg daily
Gentamicin	3mg/kg every other day
Oxytetracycline	10mg/kg daily
Potentiated sulphonamide (48%)	1ml/16kg every other day
Enrofloxacin	5-10mg/kg daily

Other drugs have been used but relatively little information is available based on controlled trials. Extrapolating from dose rates used in reptiles may be useful.

The actual route of injection is a matter of preference, and several are used. My own preference is into the dorsal sinus, situated in the midline anterior to the dorsal fin, between the two 'fillets'. Injection by this method can often be done without anaesthesia, and clinical results suggest that absorption from this site is good.

Other sites are:

1. The lateral musculature, half way between the leading edge of the dorsal fin and the lateral line.
2. The tail muscles posterior to the vent, popular with hobbyists to avoid any internal organs.

3. Intra-peritoneal, a variable distance anterior to the vent and just off the midline - depending on the size of the fish. This route has some potential problems although it is extremely popular. In cyprinids the internal organs are very adherent to each other and drugs could be injected into an organ, into mass of fat, or potentially eliminated through the abdominal pore.

It is important when injecting fish to avoid scale damage and so needles should be introduced between scales. If they are pushed through scales, great care should be taken on removal to avoid pulling the scale out.

Other licensed compounds used in fish disease treatment

Andrews and Riley (1982) used praziquantel (Droncit, Bayer) at 27.4-34.25mg/kg body weight in a successful trial to eliminate *Bothriocephalus acheilognathi* from carp (*Cyprinus carpio*), grass carp (*Ctenopharyngodon idella*), tench (*Tinca tinca*) and wels (*Silurus glanis*). Pool et al (1984), also used 35-100mg/kg (given by stomach tube) effectively and safely in grass carp infected with *Bothriocephalus acheilognathi*. A dose of 125mg/kg body weight fed over a three day period by top-dressing pelleted food also proved effective.

Hyland and Adams (1987) reported the use of ivermectin in goldfish for the treatment of anchor worm. The drug was given by injection at a dose of 200µg/kg (first diluted 1:125 with physiological saline, this then used at 0.1ml/50g by intramuscular injection at the base of the dorsal fin). They report the parasite dying and withering, with healing occurring rapidly. It is uncertain whether this treatment would eliminate the larvae on the gills. Stoskopf (1988) comments that ivermectin at 100µg/kg affects many fish before it affects the parasites.

A number of antimalarials have been used very successfully against a number of marine protozoal infections (Kingsford, 1975). Experience using chloroquine in this way in one of the newer 'complete ecosystem' tanks (dependent on the interaction between fish, invertebrates, algae and bacteria) suggests that these drugs may have disastrous effects on such aquaria by upsetting this balance (Helme, personal communication).

Levamisole has been used apparently successfully at 10mg/litre for a number of years against nematodes in fish such as livebearers infected with *Camallanus* spp. or Discus (*Symphysodon discus*) infected with *Capillaria* spp. No adverse effects have been reported and fish have bred afterwards.

Other products licensed as pesticides have been used against *Lernaea* spp and *Argulus* spp. These include trichlorphon (Dipterex 80, Bayer), diflubenzuron (Dimilin WP, ICI), bromex (Naled, Kyldane). Dichlorvos (Nuvan, Ciba Geigy) was licensed as an insecticide but due to widespread use in salmon was licensed as a medicine under the name Aquagard (Ciba Geigy). Unfortunately dose titration has not yet been carried out for its application to ornamental fish. Hopefully other compounds of this type will become available.

Because resistance to organophosphorus compounds has become noticeable among monogenea of ornamental fish, Goven and Amend (1980) reported work on combination treatments using mebendazole and trichlorphon. This resistance is particularly seen with *Gyrodactylus* spp where the dose of trichlorphon required to kill them in some cases has risen from 0.25mg/litre to 25mg/litre (toxic for fish). Mebendazole was found to be effective against *Gyrodactylus elegans* at doses of 0.1mg/litre, but had no effect on *Dactylogyrus vastator* up to 2mg/litre. Fortunately resistance in the latter is not as widespread. Because trichlorphon seems to reduce the efficacy of mebendazole, a final dose rate of 0.4mg/litre mebendazole and 1.8mg/litre trichlorphon was recommended. The minimum exposure time is 24 hours and no adverse effects have been reported on a range of ornamental fish except perhaps catfish.Successful trials were reported in goldfish (*Carassius auratus*), oscars (*Astronotus ocellatus*), angel fish (*Pterophyllum scalare*), molly (*Poecilia velifera*), and gourami (*Trichogaster trichopterus*).

Vaccines

Vaccination is only now becoming possible for ornamental fish. Vaccines against Vibrios, Enteric Redmouth and Furunculosis have been available for some time for the food-fish farmer, but strain variation has hindered their application to ornamentals. Recently Aquavac Cyprivac CE (AVL) has become available for vaccination of cyprinids (such as goldfish and koi) against erythrodermatitis or Ulcer disease caused by *Aeromonas salmonicida*. Hopefully this will reduce the problems widely seen and also herald other vaccines for SVC and Vibriosis in ornamental marine fish.

UNLICENSED COMPOUNDS USED IN FISH DISEASE TREATMENT

Benzalkonium chloride

This family of chemicals are powerful disinfectants with an additional detergent action. Benzalkonium chloride is a blend of quaternary ammonium compounds although not all such blends are suitable for use in fish treatment. It is used for certain external bacterial diseases, though is generally not as useful as chloramine T.

Benzalkonium chloride (Ark-Klens, Vetark) is particularly useful in treating external bacterial infections such as Bacterial Gill Disease (BGD) where Myxobacteria are multiplying within a film of mucus on the gills. The dual action is important since bacterial growth is inhibited and the mucus lifted off by the detergent effect. Other uses are as a disinfectant for nets where other chemicals might be dangerous, or for reducing the bacterial loading in water containing fish with bacterial diseases such as Enteric redmouth.

In rapid turnover flow-through systems (5-10 minutes) up to 10mg/litre may be needed, while with slower turnover systems (30 minutes) 5 mg/litre may be used. For bath treatment in a static system, such as a treatment tank, 1mg/litre is used for 1 hour.

In very slow earth ponds it may be necessary to use doses lower than 0.5mg/litre. In aquaria and static ponds doses between 0.1-0.5mg/litre have been used.

In flow-through systems repeat treatments are often used to relieve the signs of gill disease and aid the fishes' respiration by reducing the mucus coating. Because the compound is relatively stable. Repeat treatments should not be carried out in the domestic pond/tank situation without first carrying out major water changes to eliminate any residual benzalkonium chloride.

Broodstock may be usefully treated since the chemical also has mild antifungal properties.

The toxicity of benzalkonium chloride is increased in soft water so treatment levels should be at least halved. Where there is doubt, lower doses should be tried first and then increased as appropriate. It is reported than salmon intended for release should not be treated since the chemical inhibits the sense of smell and so can affect its ability to return to its home river.

Dose (mg/litre)	Duration of treatment
10	5-10 min
5	30 min
2	60 min
1	several hours

Chloramine-T

This is one of the more useful chemicals available to the fish keeper (Chloramine-T: Vetark). It has an effect against Myxobacteria, *Costia*, white spot and *Gyrodactylus*. The quality of the material is important as toxic complexes may be formed by impurities. This is less of a problem if the chemical is used simply as a disinfectant. It is important to avoid contact with the skin or eyes and so a mask and gloves should be used. The compound should be stored in a dry cool place and protected from sunlight.

The action of chloramine T is based on a slow breakdown to hypochlorous acid releasing oxygen and chlorine. Because of this it should not be used at the same time as any other chemicals, such as formalin or benzalkonium chloride.

The following table of doses was suggested for flow systems with a 4 hour turnover (Cross and Hursey, 1973), and where appropriate they can be repeated three times at 4 hour intervals.

Therapeutic dose (mg/litre)

pH	Soft Water	Hard water
6.0	2.5	7.0
6.5	5.0	10
7.0	10	15
7.5	18	18
8.0	20	20

In general one should always err on the side of caution and start with a 2mg/litre dose rate which can be increased carefully as necessary. Chloramine-T has been used in static systems at lower dose rates of 0.5-2mg/litre.

Copper Sulphate

Copper sulphate has been extensively used in fish, as a long standing 'traditional' dip treatment against bacterial gill disease, although this cannot be recommended in general. Its prime action is as an astringent, literally shrinking gill cells off mucus, but unfortunately this action also affects the cells of the liver.

The use of copper at a low level dose as a treatment against *Oodinium*, *Amyloodinium*, *Cryptocaryon* and a range of other protozoal infections in freshwater and marine tanks has been reviewed by Cardheilhac and Whitaker (1988).

A stock solution is prepared by dissolving 400mg $CuSO_4.5H_2O$. in 1 litre of water. This is then used at a dose of 1ml/litre. For large systems, a tenfold concentration can be made up using 4g of $CuSO_4.5H_2O$. per litre of water. The dose of the latter is 1ml/10 litres.

This dose rate gives a theoretical copper concentration of 0.1mg/litre. The actual level of free copper should be tested using a professional standard test (such as Lovibond or Hach, not hobbyist quality) and sufficient of the stock solution added to bring the level to 0.2 mg/litre. Water changes should be carried out if the level rises too high.

Daily tests should be performed so that a level of 0.1-0.2 mg/litre is maintained for at least 10 days. In freshwater, care needs to be taken since the dose depends on water hardness

Copper can be removed from the system by water changes although this takes time. For a more rapid effect, a large amount of activated carbon (approximately 3g for every litre of water being treated) can be used.

Trichlorphon

Dipterex, Dylox, and Masoten all contain trichlorphon. This can only be obtained as an insecticide and since it does not have a product licence for fish use, suppliers may refuse to supply the compound if they suspect that it is to be used as a medicine. There may be scope for other products to be used instead and perhaps future editions of this manual will be able to clarify the situation.

Trichlorphon, when added to water, breaks down to produce dichlorvos (the active chemical in terms of killing parasites). Ultimately it is thought that dichlorvos breaks down further to dimethyl hydrogen phosphate and other chemicals which are biodegradeable. This is a pH dependant breakdown with a variable time scale, slow in acid water and rapid in hard, alkaline or sea water.

It may take up to 3 weeks in acid water.

pH	1/2 life at 20-23°C
7	21 days
9	1 day

It has been used widely in both fresh and salt water as a fish ectoparasiticide, to kill a number of the larger parasites such as Flukes, *Argulus* (fish lice) and *Lernaea* (Anchor worms). Claims of efficacy against protozoa are uncertain. Resistance has now been reported (Goven, et al. 1980).

It is generally used at concentrations of:
    0.2 mg/litre active ingredient as a permanent treatment.
    2-2.5% dip. This has been used for cyprinids for up to 5-10 minutes.

In general its use as a dip should be cautioned against. It is dangerous to handle and very easily causes damage to fish (such as broken backs from convulsing). To dispose of the dip, add 8g of caustic soda per 10g of trichlorphon used and leave for 6 hours before pouring to waste.

The use of repeat treatments will need to be based on water chemistry (as above). Weekly treatments in hard water areas appear to be the norm, whilst in soft water these may be too frequent. In marine tanks, treatment every 3 days is commonly used.

Treating new species should be done with caution as there appear to be some species which are highly susceptible to its toxic effects.

Trichlorphon is toxic to orfe (*Leuciscus idus*), chubb (*Leuciscus cephalus*) & rudd (*Scardinius erythrophthalmus*) and possibly also to golden tench (*Tinca tinca*), although green tench (*Tinca tinca*) have not shown problems. Characins, in general, are sensitive. Toxicity to other fish and higher animals is relatively low and its highest toxicity is towards invertebrates, in particular crustacea.

Formalin

Formalin is used for the treatment of ectoparasitic infections of fish, particularly those caused by protozoa (eg. *Costia, Trichodina, Chilodonella*). It is also effective against the monogenetic skin and gill flukes (eg. *Dactylogyrus* and *Gyrodactylus*)

The normal treatment level is:
    1:6000 (167mg/litre) - 1:4000 (250mg/litre) for up to 1 hour
This is equivalent to 1 ml of 40% formaldehyde in 4.55 litres of water for up to 1 hour.

It is also used at a dose of 2 drops of 40% formaldehyde in 4.55 litres of water as a permanent bath.

In most cases, the lower level is preferred although the high dose may be required if it is being used against *Epistylis* or *Chilodonella*, particularly with pond fish at low temperatures. *Chilodonella* infections are often in fact resistant to other treatments.

The dip should be aerated during use, and it should be observed all the time so that fish can be removed if they show signs of distress. Formalin is a reducing agent and toxicity may be seen during the course of treatment or for up to 24 hours afterwards. Fish with gill disease or anaemia should only be treated with great caution because formalin has an astringent effect which literally shrinks the cells of the gill. Repeat treatments are to be avoided since both the gills and liver suffer damage which may be cumulative.

Formalin must be fresh, and if any precipitate of paraformaldehyde is present this must be filtered out prior to use.

Leteux-Meyer mixture

This term was used by Scott (1982) to describe the mixture of formalin and malachite green tested by these authors (Leteux and Meyer, 1972). There are several variations on the basic combination of chemicals which originally aimed to give a treatment dose of 25mg/litre formalin and 0.05 mg/litre of malachite green.

One common formulation is made by adding 3.68g of malachite green to one litre of formalin. This is used at a rate of 25mg/litre formalin (plus 0.05mg/litre malachite green) for 1 hour. There have been a number of 'over-the-counter' products available containing mixtures of formalin and malachite green at various levels, usually formulated to be used over a five day period. These are all in a "statutory limbo" at present while the legislation is being clarified.

In static ponds a weaker mixture of 3.3g of malachite green in 1 litre of formalin can be used at a dose of 15mg/litre formalin (plus 0.05mg/litre malachite green). If necessary it may be used at 3-4 day intervals, providing that dissolved oxygen levels remain above 5 mg/litre and the temperature below 28°C.

In static systems with coldwater fish it has proved effective against a wide range if protozoa, including white spot. In most cases just a single treatment is used, although, where problems are severe, further treatments can be carried out if felt necessary. Treatment on two consecutive days has proved to be safe (Scott, unpublished data) but then water changes need to be carried out to avoid toxicity from the malachite green. Lack of green colouration is no indication of the absence of the latter since it may simply be a chemical change to the colourless form. Clients should always be warned to be aware of possible adverse reactions, and advised to carry out immediate major water changes should any problems be suspected.

Malachite green

This is used for treatment of fungal infections, and when mixed with formalin, for the treatment of protozoal infections (see Leteux Meyer mixture).

When treating eggs of fish against fungal infections it is usually used as a 2mg/litre flowing treatment for 30-60 minutes.

Commonly used dosages are;

    Dose: -   2 mg/litre for 30 min
                0.1 mg/litre as a permanent bath

Toxicity may appear as respiratory distress. This is usually immediate rather then delayed, and is likely to be irreversible since malachite green affects the cytochrome oxidase system.

Traditionally one would advise the use of the zinc free form of malachite green, although this is still no guarantee of safety. Malachite green is toxic to tetras and some other small characins and scaleless fish. A detailed review of malachite green has been carried out by Alderman (1985).

Salt

Sodium chloride is one of the longest standing aquarium treatments (Mulertt, 1902). I has been widely used as an osmotic support for stressed or sick fish, and to reduce gill mucus in fish with compromised gills. Salt is also very valuable as a part of the treatment of ulcers, by reducing the osmotic gradient between the fish and its surroundings the bed of the ulcer remains viable longer and stands a better chance of healing. The gills of freshwater fish actively take up salt from the water, and the greater the osmotic gradient the more energy must be expended. Maintaining fish in saline solutions thus significantly decreases the amount of metabolic effort required for the fish to maintain physiological homeostasis. (McWilliams, personal communication).

For treatment of fish to reduce osmotic stress a level of 0.15% (1500 mg/litre) on day 1, can be built up to 0.6% (3000 mg/litre) over 3 days. If any signs of distress are seen the solution should be diluted and a slower increase used. The majority of carp will tolerate an immediate transfer to a saline solution but a gradual increase in salt level is less of a shock.

Alevins and small fry can be treated with 0.5% (5000 mg/litre) for 30 minutes, or 1% (10,000 mg/litre) for 6-10 minutes. Larger fish may be given progressively larger doses such that fish larger than 300g can be treated with 3% salt (30,000 mg/litre) for about 2 minutes or until they show signs of distress.

As a general rule it is recommended that alevins and fry under 100/lb (5g) should not be exposed to over 1% (10,000 mg/litre) sodium chloride, and that fish under 5/lb should not be exposed to levels greater than 2% (20,000 mg/litre).

Another treatment which has been found effective in very large volume systems where true salting would not be feasible is to cross-cut 25kg salt bags and tether them in the shallows, or to place heaps of salt in tanks. Fish with excess mucus on their gills will follow the salt concentration and dose themselves, often almost swimming into the bag (Scott, unpublished data).

Potassium permanganate

Potassium permanganate has been used as a treatment for protozoal and monogenean parasites, bacterial gill disease (BGD) and oxygen depletion. Its use requires careful observation and effort to devise regimes which are both safe and effective, and in general it should not be recommended. In muddy water it may be neutralised totally and rendered ineffective, and it may lead to toxic effects due to the deposition of manganese dioxide on the gills. Care needs to be taken in warm water and with scaleless fish such as eels.

For the treatment of BGD it has been used at 1-5mg/litre for 1 hour, repeating as necessary for 2-3 days. An alternative means of administration is by short duration (10-40 seconds) dip treatment in a 1000 mg/litre solution. As an emergency procedure in static ponds it has been used for treatment of oxygen depletion at a dose of 2mg/litre.

Phenoxyethanol

This has been used at a concentration of 0.1-0.5ml/litre (100-500mg/litre) as an anaesthetic. It also has bactericidal effects and may therefore be of some use when handling broodstock in reducing surface contamination. As an antibacterial it has been sold for aquarium use since 1955 (Yates, 1955). There is an increased safety margin at lower temperatures since the lower doses can be used.

The lower level (0.1 ml/litre) is reported useful for prolonged sedation. At a concentration of 1ml/litre (1000mg/litre) it gives rapid anaesthesia and fish must be removed quickly when anaesthetised or they will die.

Care needs to be taken when advising its use. I is reported to elute toxins from activated carbon in filters.

Methylene Blue

This has been in use for many years at a concentration of between 1-2mg/litre as an antiprotozoal treatment. It is extremely harmful to biological filter systems and for this reason should not be used in recirculation systems without taking precautions for treatment off-circuit or stripping the system down after treatment and re-establishing the filter.

Another potential use is as an emergency treatment for nitrite toxicity. Here the aim is to convert methaemoglobin back to haemoglobin, and in salmon it has been used at around 1mg/litre.

PRACTICAL TREATMENT/CONTROL REGIMES

Ulcer disease

Unfortunately the misuse of antibiotics has rendered many infectious organisms resistant to treatment with "standard" antibiotics. Injections of antibiotics are of value in treating cases where this is commercially worthwhile; baths are generally not worth the cost and are generally ineffective. Various antibiotics have been used, including potentiated sulphonamides (Trivetrin & Tribrissen, Pitman-Moore), neomycin, oxytetracycline (Terramycin, Pfizer) but efficacy will depend on resistance, the stage of the disease and the overall condition of the fish under treatment.

Care must be taken with nets to avoid transmitting the disease between batches. Netting a fish with an ulcer contaminates the net, and then when used again this net rubs the organisms into the skin of another fish. Disinfection of nets using benzalkonium chloride solution is well worthwhile since it is also a detergent and lifts mucus off which might protect bacteria from the effects of a disinfectant.

The ulcers once produced take some time to heal, even once the cause has been treated and eliminated. Treatment requires anaesthesia (see chapter 18) after which vigorous cleaning and debriding of the ulcer using antibacterials such as povidone iodine (Tamodine, Vetark) on cotton wool can be performed. The bed of the ulcer can be packed using Orabase (Squibb), and antibacterials can be mixed with this if considered appropriate. This product is worked into the ulcer using wet fingers.

Fig 1 (a):
Thoroughly debride ulcer

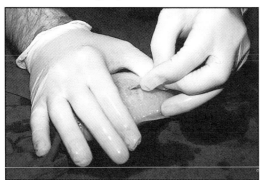

Photo: Ray Butcher

Fig 1 (b):
Clean with povidone iodine

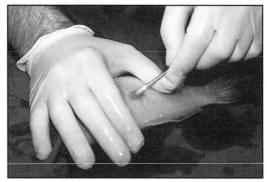

Photo: Ray Butcher

Fig 1 (c):
Pack ulcer with orabase (possibly mixed with antibacterial preps)

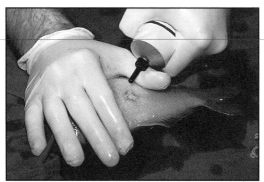

Photo: Ray Butcher

Fig 1 (d):
Inject appropriate antibiotic

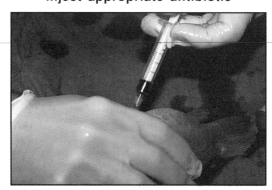

Photo: Ray Butcher

Once the ulcer has been treated, the fish is best allowed to recover and held in a salt bath (approximately 0.5%). Ulcers should be cleaned this way only once, since repeated treatments simply inhibit epithelialisation. The Orabase may remain visible for up to 2 weeks. In general repeated handling of fish even for 'necessary' treatment is stressful and to be avoided. Even with summer temperatures several weeks are needed to allow time to heal and particularly with goldfish or small koi this can be uneconomic for the retailer or wholesaler and considered bad economic sense. A severe outbreak under such circumstances may be best treated by destruction of stock and subsequent disinfection.

Anchor worm (*Lernaea* spp) infection

Infections with this parasite need to take into account the life cycle. Adult parasites are very resistant to treatment and need individual attention. Fish are anaesthetised and examined behind the fins, on the body, and under opercula etc for the presence of *Lernaea*. If found, they should be gently but firmly grasped using forceps and pulled out, ensuring that the 'anchor' is extracted. The hole remaining is then treated as an ulcer. The work using ivermectin (see Other licensed products) may be very promising in this regard since the parasites seem to have been killed in situ and quickly shrivelled and allowed healing around them.

It is crucial with this infection to treat the water in which fish are held with an organophosphate (or other suitable compound). This is necessary to kill any larvae which are on the gills of the fish. (see chapter 9)

CHAPTER TWENTY TWO

QUARANTINE

Chris Andrews
Ray L Butcher

GENERAL CONSIDERATIONS

The quarantining of all new fish and plants is very important to prevent the introduction of diseases into already established aquaria and ponds. Apparently healthy fish can carry a huge range of disease organisms as sub-clinical infections. These infections are often extremely difficult to detect, yet may wreak havoc when introduced into the relatively overcrowded confines of a pond or aquarium. Even with carefully chosen fish from a reputable dealer, there is still a risk of introducing potentially dangerous pathogens, and this is often overlooked.

Recently imported fish that have, by the very nature of the trade, already undergone a period of severe stress and overstocking, are especially dangerous in this respect. The trigger factors necessary to set off a disease outbreak in these fish may already have occurred, but the associated clinical signs may not become apparent for several weeks due to the sometimes relatively long incubation periods involved.

A further factor worthy of consideration is the apparent misunderstanding amongst some traders/ hobbyists of what the term "quarantine" actually means. Some may feel that a day or so is all that is required, while others fail to completely isolate the fish at all. In such cases, the period of "quarantine" is synonymous simply with the time between the arrival of the fish on the premises, and resale. This may not be commonplace, but it highlights the importance of careful history taking.

The quarantine period should be for at least four weeks, and during that time the new fish should be kept completely separate from all others. To avoid transferring disease organisms, it is important to have a complete set of equipment (such as nets, buckets, scrapers, siphon tube etc.) exclusively for use in the quarantine tank. Furthermore, any routine maintenance on the quarantine tank should be carried out after, and never before, attending to the main aquarium or pond. Personal hygiene is also important, as fish disease organisms can be carried on wet hands. During quarantine, the fish should be observed closely for any unusual symptoms or behaviour. It is much easier to deal with any signs of disease in the quarantine tank than in a set-up aquarium or pond. Even if the fish seem healthy it is probably a good idea to give them a preventative course of treatment with an appropriate anti-parasite remedy.

Generally speaking, low temperatures slow down the life cycles of most fish pathogens such that any symptoms of disease take longer to show. Ideally, tropical fish should be quarantined at 72-77°F (22-25°C) and cold water fish at no less than 54-59°F (12-15°C). At lower temperatures, it is best to at least double the often-quoted four week quarantine period.

If, after four weeks, the quarantined fish have shown no signs of disease, they can be carefully introduced into the set-up aquarium or pond. Even then, however, they are still unlikely to be pathogen-free. Latent infections may remain in or on their bodies, which highlights the importance of correct care in enhancing their natural resistance and thus preventing outbreaks of disease.

Aquarium fish

It is relatively simple to set up a quarantine tank for aquarium fish and small pond fish. All that is required is a small to medium sized tank with a lid (10-20 gallons or 45-90 litres is fine), a foam cartridge filter run from an air pump or a small internal power filter, a heater-thermostat for tropical fish, a thermometer and one or two plastic plants or half flower pots to act as refuges for the fish. A fairly spartan tank will make cleaning after quarantining each batch of fish much easier.

To provide biologically mature water, either keep the quarantine tank ticking over with a couple of hardy fishes, such as mollies or goldfish, or try to use a foam cartridge or filter medium which has been used previously in the main tank with a fish population. For marine fish, it is particularly important that the quarantine tank is a miniature version of the full set up, preferably using fully mature filters to minimise the stress on the new fish.

Pond fish

In order to quarantine all but the smallest pond fish, one would need larger facilities than those described. A large aquarium (at least 30 gallons or 135 litres) will suffice in some instances; other receptacles such as children's paddling pools, or a large cardboard box lined with a polythene liner can be pressed into service at short notice. Whatever is used, it is important to cover the container with a fine-meshed nylon net, stretched tight and weighted down. This will keep the fish in and children, cats and birds out. Filtration is probably not required for most pond fish, although aeration is very important, particularly during warm weather. Avoid direct sunlight if quarantining fish in the garden.

Plants

If they have come from an environment inhabited by fish, plants may also introduce pests and diseases. Ideally therefore wash new plants in lukewarm water and quarantine them in a fish-free tank at room temperature for several days. A more specific way of dealing with any pathogens present is to treat the plants with a plant disinfectant or mild broad spectrum anti-parasite remedy during their quarantine period.

Prophylactic Treatments

Since all new fish are a potential source of disease organisms, it might seem sensible to treat them with some broad spectrum medication(s) during the quarantine period. However, many of the commonly used antibacterial and antiparasitic agents may themselves be toxic to the gills (Chapters 13 and 21). If the fish have been stressed, or kept in overcrowded conditions immediately prior to the quarantine period (e.g: recently imported fish), it is likely that the gill function is already severely compromised. Treatment with these agents early on during the quarantine period could therefore be disasterous.

The prime consideration in such circumstances is to keep the fish in as stress free an environment as possible with optimum water quality conditions. As mentioned in Chapter 2, the optimum water quality conditions will vary with the species involved. For freshwater fish it may be of benefit to add salt to the water, as this will reduce the osmotic gradient across the gills, and hence decrease the fish's energy requirements (Chapter 21).

Antibacterial or antiparasitic treatments are best deferred for a couple of weeks. The choice of the agent used will reflect the efficacy and toxicity of the compound in the particular water quality conditions appropriate for the species of fish concerned (Chapter 21), as well as the nature of the infective organism thought to pose the greatest risk. In a large shipment of fish, the sampling of a representative sample on arrival may be of use in this respect.

Antibiotics may be of value when specifically indicated by the clinical signs. These, however, are best given incorporated in the feed rather than added to the water (Chapter 21), and the agent used is of necessity often chosen on the basis of an 'educated guess' rather than on specific sensitivity patterns. Bacteria recovered from recently imported fish may exhibit fairly broad antibiotic resistance due in part to their widespread use in the Far East.

CHAPTER TWENTY THREE

LEGAL ASPECTS

Peter W Scott

This chapter is written from the standpoint of a practising veterinary surgeon, rather than that of a member of the legal profession. Much of the law relating to fish has not truly been challenged, or even clarified, and there are serious problem areas, notably the perception of pain and the concept of suffering. For a strict legal interpretation the appropriate references should be read.

The Veterinary Surgeons Act, 1966

It is worth noting that for the purposes of this Act the definition of "animals" includes birds and reptiles but not fish. This doesn't quite leave a free-for-all, however, since fish included in other legislation, particularly:

The Medicines Act, 1968
Protection of Animals Act, 1911

The Guide to Professional Conduct Section 1.5 makes clear the responsibility of a veterinary surgeon to provide emergency first aid for all species and to ensure that the client can reach more experienced help. He, personally, should make contact with another colleague who can deal with the case. In circumstances where no practice in an area has the necessary expertise, the RCVS makes it clear that practices must take all reasonable steps to obtain assistance so that the public (and the animals) are not denied help. It is not acceptable to fob off a client with the telephone number of a veterinary surgeon 50 or 350 miles away. Generally, those in 'fish' practice are usually more than willing to advise colleagues directly.

The Medicines Act 1968

This Act, strangely perhaps in the light of the Veterinary Surgeons Act,(1966) does include fish. Hence POM products may be prescribed only for animals under the care of a veterinary surgeon. The question of at what stage a tank of fish realistically comes 'under ones care' is open to discussion, and whether examining one cadaver brought to the surgery is sufficient, or whether a site visit is required may vary with circumstances.

The vast majority of treatments used for ornamental fish are currently unlicensed as medicines. Traditionally these have been sold through pet shops and garden centres etc, and many of these outlets may also give advice regarding fish. This has not been ideal but it is extremely unlikely that most of these products will be licensed and although the European Community (E.C.) has looked at exemption schemes for these products (EC Directive /881/EEC serra 4), these have not been adopted in the UK as yet. This leaves veterinary surgeons etc. in a dilemma regarding the stocking and the use of unlicensed medicines, since to do otherwise may itself cause welfare problems. Hopefully, this situation may be resolved in the near future.

A further problem is that many fish outlets sell chemicals which in another guise are licensed drugs (eg benzocaine). The law here has also been rather vague. Benzocaine, for example, becomes an anaesthetic (and hence a licensed drug) only when the customer chooses to use it as such. Hopefully this anomalous situation will also be resolved.

The Veterinary Surgeons Act 1966 (Schedule 3 Amendment) Order 1988

This amendment changes the type of treatment which can be carried out on animals (as covered by the 1966 Act) by the owner. It therefore makes no reference to fish.

Protection of Animals Act, 1911 (1912 Scotland)

This Act deals with the subject of unnecessary suffering. It states that:

1.1 If any person-

a) shall cruelly beat, kick, ill-treat, over-ride, over drive, over-load, torture, infuriate, or terrify any animal, or shall cause or procure, or, being the owner, permit any animal to be so used, or shall, by wantonly or unreasonably doing or omitting to do any act, or causing or procuring the commission or omission of any act, cause any unnecessary suffering, or, being the owner, permit any unnecessary suffering to be so caused to any animal; or

b) shall convey or carry, or cause or procure, or, being the owner, permit to be conveyed or carried, any animal in such manner or position as to cause that animal any unnecessary suffering,...etc

such person shall be guilty of an offence of cruelty within the meaning of this Act,... etc

Cooper (1987) has discussed the implications of this in detail, and explains that to show that an offence under section one has been committed, it is necessary to show that an act both causes suffering and that it was unnecessary. It also needs to be unreasonable and, by case law, 'substantial'.

The above is of significance in relation to whether fish suffer or feel pain. Although difficult to argue, there is considerable evidence to support the premis and little to refute it. The Government commissioned "Report of the Panel of Enquiry into Shooting and Angling" (1976-1979) recommended that "where considerations of welfare are involved, all vertebrate animals (ie. mammals, birds, amphibians and fish) should be regarded as equally capable of suffering to some degree or another, without distinction between "warm-blooded' and "cold-blooded" species.

The Protection of Animals (Anaesthetics) Acts, 1954 and 1964

These Acts specifically exclude fish. Cooper (1983) speculates that this may be because satisfactory methods of anaesthesia were not envisaged at that time. It is likely, however, that suffering resulting from failure to use an anaesthetic where appropriate, would be regarded as and offence under the Protection of Animals Act, 1911.

Import of Live Fish (England and Wales) Act ,1980

This Act provides for the licensing of the importation, release or keeping of non-indigenous fish and licenses for the importation of ornamental fish have been granted freely to date, although changes being examined in the EC may alter this.

Diseases of Fish Act, 1937

This Act is very important and has various significant areas of interest.

1. It deals with restrictions on the importation of live fish and eggs of fish. All fish importations require a license under this Act.

2. Contraventions result in seizure and detention of the fish or eggs. It also gives the power to designate infected areas and so can prohibit or regulate the movement of live fish or foodstuffs from that site. This takes the form of a renewable 16 day order. The occupier is entitled, on application, to a report of the evidence on which the order was made. The Minister can direct the occupier regarding removal of dead or dying fish and their disposal. This is covered in Section 2, subsection 4 and appears to exclude non fish farms (although under the Act's definition Fish dealers are fish farms).

3. The Act requires "any person entitled to take fish from any inland water, or employed for the purpose of having the care of inland waters" to report any suspected notifiable diseases to the Minister - in actuality to his agents (ie. the Ministry of Agriculture Fisheries and Food). Denham 1990, reports that the current view from MAFFs legal department is that this obligation does not extend to a veterinarian asked to examine/screen fish. However, MAFF would expect the veterinarian to advise the farmer of his obligation to report such findings.

4. If the Minister believes that any direction is not being complied with he can direct an inspector to carry it out, and then recover the cost from the occupier by civil proceedings.

5. The Minister can authorise the occupier to remove fish from an infected area if he believes it to be appropriate in the general interest. This only applies to fish farms and it authorises removal rather than requires removal.

Diseases of Fish Act, 1983

1. This modifies "infected area" to "designated area" and extends the controls to prohibiting the taking into or out of the area live fish or eggs or foodstuff for fish. It changes the 16 day order to 30 days, and this can then be extended to 60 days and further renewed. Although there are no powers of compulsory slaughter, this can be applied to ornamental fish dealers to prevent sale of live fish until the infected fish (normally all of the fish on the premises at the time) are slaughtered and the premises are disinfected satisfactorily.

2. It updates the definition of fish farm to: "any pond, stew, fish hatchery or other place used for keeping, with a view to their sale or to their transfer to other waters (including any other fish farm) live fish, live eggs of fish, or foodstuffs for fish, and includes any buildings used in connection therewith, and the banks and margins of any water therein;" and refers to the "business of fish farming" as meaning "business of keeping live fish (whether or not for profit) with a view to their sale or to their transfer to other waters". This widens the definition and essentially brings ornamental retailers, wholesalers and many hobbyists who breed and sell, within the Act.

3. It requires registration of the fish farm and requires submissions relating to stock movements

The Minister has the right to add diseases to the list of those covered by the provisions of the Diseases of Fish Acts (1937 & 1983).

Zoo Licensing Act, 1981

This Act in its definitions includes all places where fish are displayed to the public. This could range from a conventional zoo to a restaurant. In practice the majority of small commercial situations where fish are used for decoration (ie shops and restaurants) are exempted by simply not being asked to register. Some have been specifically exempted where there are a number of tanks and their case merited inspection. This Act is primarily concerned with public safety, although animal welfare issues have been brought within its influence.

Pet Animals Act, 1951 and Pet Animals Act, 1951 (Amendment) Act 1982

Shops selling fish are included within the remit of this Act although its terms are relatively loose. BVA has Guidelines for Inspections under the Pet Animals Act. Local authority consultative groups are examining proposals for water standards in ornamental fish outlets prepared by Ornamental Fish Industry (UK). These will suggest minimum water quality parameters and make suggestions how they might be achieved.

Other areas considered out of the scope of this chapter but which might be relevant under certain circumstances are:

Animals (Scientific Procedures) Act,1986, which in addition to work in the laboratory regulates such procedures as fin clipping and tagging of wild fish.

Abandonment of Animals Act, 1960 makes it an offence of cruelty under the 1911 Act to abandon an animal without reasonable excuse in circumstances likely to cause it suffering. Although intended to apply to abandoned pets this might also apply to release of captive bred animals into the wild, such as restocking a river or lake with brown or rainbow trout. In 1991 the RSPCA brought a successful prosecution of an ornamental fish wholesaler under the provisions of this Act (RSPCA v.Durier 1991).

HEALTH AND SAFETY

As with all aspects of Veterinary work, Health & Safety issues are covered by the following:

Health and Safety at Work Act (1974)

Control of Pollution Act (1974)

Waste Collection and Disposal Regulations (1987)

Control of Substances Hazardous to Health Regulations (1989)

The special application to ornamental fish can be summarised as follows:

1. The use of chemicals/COSHH Regulations.

   The supply of medications to treat small numbers of fish may often require dispensing minute quantities of chemicals. The appropriate precautions should be taken if this involves staff measuring out the concentrated forms of toxic agents (especially formalin and malachite green).

   Some chemicals are supplied as a powder that requires accurate weighing before dispensing (e.g. Tricholorphon). Care should be taken to provide adequate protection from inhalation or irritation of the eyes.

2. Zoonoses.

   Mycobacterium marinum spp. has been associated with a hypersensitivity reaction on the skin of humans (the so-called "swimming pool granuloma"). This should be taken into consideration when formulating a Practice COSHH assessment.

3. Cadavers and samples from fish are classified as clinical waste and should be disposed of in the appropriate manner.

Chris Andrews

Diet
- A balanced, varied diet based on good quality dried foods.
- Avoid overfeeding.
- Use only safe live foods.

Temperature
- Avoid sudden changes.
- 73-79°F (23-26°C) for most tropical species.

Compatibility
- Ensure that all fish and/or invertebrates in the same tank will mix.
- Ensure there are refuges for timid species.
- Keep most freshwater fish in pairs or small shoals.

Stocking Level
- Coldwater aquaria: allow 24 sq.in. of water surface for each inch of fish.
- Tropical freshwater aquaria: allow 10 sq.in. of water surface for each inch of fish
- Coldwater and tropical marine aquaria: allow 60 sq.in. of water surface for each inch of fish.
- Ponds: allow 1 sq.ft. of water surface for each 2-3 inches of fish.

Note that fish over 2 inches in length will require even more space.

pH
- Avoid sudden changes.
- pH 6.5 - 7.5 is satisfactory for most freshwater fish, and 8.0 - 8.3 is satisfactory for most marine species.

Specific Gravity
- 1.020 - 1.024 for most marine organisms.
- 1.002 - 1.010 for brackish water fish.
- Always use a reliable marine salt mix.

Ammonia, Nitrite and Nitrate
- Negligible ammonia and nitrite in established tanks and ponds.
- Nitrate-nitrogen less than 20 mg per litre for delicate marine fish and invertebrates.
- Nitrate is less important for hardy marines and most freshwater fish.

Filtration and Aeration
- Ensure adequate filtration and/or aeration at all times.
- Carry out regular filter maintenance.

Partial Water Changes
- In freshwater and marine aquaria, about 25% of the tank volume should be removed every two to four weeks and topped up with conditioned water of similar temperature and quality.
- In ponds, 25% of the volume should be removed once or twice a year by trickling a hose into the pond and letting the excess overflow.

APPENDIX TWO
Glossary of Fishkeeping Terms

Chris Andrews

Actinic Tubes:

Actinic 03 lighting tubes produce light of a relatively narrow spectral quality with a peak close to the blue chlorophyll absorption peak. As a result, this type of lighting is said to be particularly beneficial for the zooanthellae within many tropical marine invertebrates.

Activated Carbon:

This is a material used in mechanical and chemical filtration systems to remove, by adsorption, various dissolved materials. Activated carbon may also function as a biological filter material after prolonged use.

Algae:

These are primitive unicellular plants and may appear in a number of forms, including phytoplankton, filamentous algae and marine macro-algae.

Biological Filtration:

This is the process by which aerobic bacteria convert nitrogenous waste material from ammonia to nitrite to nitrate.

Breeding Tank:

A tank set aside for the sole purpose of breeding fish. It is often set up along fairly spartan lines to help with cleaning, and where special attention may be paid to the specific water quality conditions required in order to induce breeding.

Community Tank:

A tank set up to contain a range of fish and perhaps plants. Care must be exercised in the choice of fish so that compatibility problems do not result.

New Tank Syndrome:

This is the characteristic rise and fall in ammonia and nitrite levels in a newly established aquarium which can be dangerous for the resident fish. Once the tank filter or filters have become colonized by aerobic bacteria, biological filtration should prevent high levels of nitrite and ammonia from occurring.

Macro-algae:

These include so-called marine "plants" such as *Caulerpa* which, despite their appearance, are actually algae rather than higher plants.

Mechanical Filtration:

This is the process by which the filter medium or media remove suspended particulate matter from the pond or aquarium water. As a result of this activity, mechanical filters will of course become clogged with this debris with time and therefore must be cleaned or the medium or media renewed.

Ozone:

This is the three-atom unstable form of oxygen which can be used as a disinfectant, and to improve the efficiency of protein skimmers in salt-water. It must be used with care as it can be toxic to fish, invertebrates and humans. Used at a low level, it will also remove colour from aquarium water.

Photosynthesis:

This is the process by which plants under bright light take-up carbon dioxide and give off oxygen as they build up simple carbohydrates within their tissues.

Protein Skimming:

This process, which is carried out by a protein skimmer, removes protein material from salt water. Protein skimmers may be air-operated or electrical water-pump powered.

Reverse-Flow Undergravel Filtration:

This process draws water from the aquarium, mechanically filters it via an external or internal power filter before forcing the water down the uplift tube of an undergravel filter and then up through the bed of gravel on the aquarium floor. Since the water is pre-filtered, the gravel bed on the aquarium floor stays cleaner for much longer when compared to ordinary undergravel filtration.

Species Tank:

This is a tank set up for the maintenance and often breeding of a single species of fish and takes account of its special environment and water quality preferences.

Tap Water Conditioners:

These may be purchased from aquarium shops to remove chlorine and some other potentially toxic substances from tap water. Some are also said to "age" new water thus making it more suitable for fishkeeping.

Ultraviolet Irradiation:

Special units produce light of a particular wave length that can be used to disinfect aquarium water. Water must be passed through these units using a water pump and it is important not to look at an operating UV lamp without protective goggles. Like any such lighting tube, UV tubes will require regular replacement if they are to perform effectively. Some success has also been achieved in the use of UV irradiation in the control of algal blooms in garden ponds.

Venturi Device:

This is a simple valve-like device used to introduce air into water as it passes along a pipe.

Zeolite:

This is a chemical filtration medium which removes nitrites and ammonia from freshwater aquaria and ponds. Its activity will become exhausted after a while, whereupon it can be recharged by soaking in a concentrated salt solution for several hours.

Zooxanthellae:

These are symbiotic single celled algae with a yellow brown pigment which live in the body cells of many protozoans, coelenterates and certain other invertebrates. Like plants, they photosynthesize in bright light and the products of this process are useful to their host organisms.

Anchor Worm	:	caused by the parasite *Lernaea* sp.
Black Spot	:	caused by larval stages of digenetic fluke parasites.
Carp Pox	:	viral infection by ? Herpes virus
Cichlid Bloat	:	synonym for Malawi Bloat
Coral Fish Disease	:	synonym for Velvet Disease
Cotton Wool Disease	:	caused by the bacterium *Cytophaga* sp. (*Flexibacter* sp.) (also called Mouth Fungus)
Dropsy	:	ascites / swollen abdomen
Eye Fluke	:	caused by larval stages of digenetic fluke parasites.
Fin Rot	:	caused by a variety of bacteria, including *Aeromonas* sp., *Pseudomonas* sp., and myxobacteria.
Fish Lice	:	infestation by the parasite *Argulus* sp.
Fish Maggots	:	infestation by the parasite *Ergasilus* sp.
Gas bubble Disease	:	supersaturation of nitrogen or oxygen
Gill Rot	:	bacterial gill disease
Gill Fluke	:	infestation principally by the parasite *Dactylogyrus* sp.
Gold Dust Disease	:	synonym for Velvet Disease
Guppy Disease	:	infection by *Tetrahymena Corlissi*.
Hole in the Head Disease	:	principally a disease of cichlids gouramis. Infection by *Hexamita* sp. thought to be involved.
Ich	:	caused by the parasite *Ichthyophthirius multifiliis* (also called "White Spot")
Malawi Bloat	:	infection by *Cryptobia* Sp.
Mouth Fungus	:	caused by the bacterium *Cytophaga* sp. (*Flexibacter* sp.) (also called Cotton Wool Disease)
Neon Tetra Disease	:	infection by *Pleistophora hyphessobryconis*
Nodular Disease	:	caused by infestation by a variety of microsporidian and myxosporidian parasites.
Pop-eye	:	exophthalmos, often occurring along with Dropsy
Rust	:	synonym for Velvet disease
Skin Fluke	:	infestation principally by the parasite *Gyrodactylus* sp.
Slime Disease	:	an excess of skin mucus produced in response to irritation by whatever cause
Swimbladder Disease	:	fish shows difficulty in maintaining its position in the water - often due to stress (c.f. the specific viral disease of Swimbladder Inflammation, (S.B.I.)
TET disease	:	synonym for Guppy Killer
Ulcer Disease	:	caused by a variety of bacteria, including *Aeromonas* sp., *Pseudomonas* sp. and *Vibrio* sp.
Velvet Disease	:	infestation by *Amyloodinium* sp. or *Oodinium* sp.
White Spot	:	caused by the parasite *Ichthyophthirius multifiliis* (also called "Ich")

E Branson
P Southgate

Some of the most obvious findings in 'sick' fish are listed below, along with some of the possible differential diagnoses. This is by no means a comprehensive list and is only intended to give an idea of possible causes.

The various presenting signs have been considered under the following headings:

1. Behavioural changes.
2. Skin problems.
3. Fin problems.
4. Eye problems.
5. Gill problems.
6. General signs visible externally.
7. Internal changes.

1. Behavioural Changes

Symptom	Possible Causes
'Gasping' at water surface, crowding at water inlet.	- Low oxygen levels. - Impaired oxygen uptake (e.g: associated with gill damage or anaemia).
'Flashing' - sudden darting through the water showing the paler underside.	- External irritation (e.g: due to parasites or waterborne irritants).
Rubbing	- As for 'flashing'
Fin clamping - where this is abnormal for the species.	- As for 'flashing'
'Coughing' material	- Presence of excess mucus or extraneous on the gills.
Lethargy, inappetence, colour changes and behavioural abnormalities.	- General debilitating illness of any cause.
Sudden death of several fish with no symptoms	- Low oxygen levels just before dawn (especially affects large fish). - peracute bacterial infections. - toxic gases from sediment due to, for example, pond cleaning. - other exogenous toxins.

2. Skin Problems

Symptom	Possible Cause
Loss and/or changes in colour	- Excess mucus production, - debilitating disease - Neon Tetra disease
Gold or rust coloured velvety patches	- Velvet disease
Small white spots on skin	- 'Ich'
Large white 'candle-wax' spots on skin.	- Carp Pox
Whitish patches on skin tissue	- Tet disease - physical damage with swelling and oedema.
Whitish 'cotton wool'-like patches	- *Epistylis* sp. - Saprolegniasis - 'myxobacteria'
Black spots on skin	- Infection with *Neascus* sp.
Black patches on skin	- Melanoma
Excess mucus on skin	- Irritant in water - ectoparasites - infection with 'myxobacteria'.
Swellings in or just below the skin.	- Parasitic cysts (e.g: due to myxosporidia, nematode larvae, digenean trematodes, etc.) - Tet disease. - Granulomata of any cause. - Fibromata and other tumours.
'Growths' on skin	- Tumours (e.g: papilloma) - viral infections (e.g: carp pox and lymphocystis)
Scale haemorrhages, petechiation.	- Viral infections - Acute bacterial infections - vitamin deficiencies.
Haemorrhagic skin damage	- Skin irritation resulting in rubbing. - direct result of ectoparasites - endoparasites just below the skin - sunburn - mechanical damage resulting from birds, handling, violent spawning behaviour.
Skin ulcers	- Secondary bacterial infection of any damaged areas (see haemorrhagic skin damage) - acute and chronic bacterial infections - Tet disease - 'Hole-in -the-Head' disease - ruptured granulomata or tumours.
Small bubbles in skin	- Gas bubble disease (also present behind the eye).

3. Fin Problems

Symptoms	Possible Causes
Ragged and damaged fins	- Ectoparasites - 'myxobacterial' infections - gas bubble disease - nutritional deficiency.
Fin haemorrhages	- See scale haemorrhages

4. Eye Problems

Symptom	Possible Causes
Blindness (Corneal opacity)	- water quality problems - mechanical damage - internal damage due to 'eye flukes' - chronic supersaturation - nutritional cataract
Small bubbles behind eye	- Gas bubble disease.
Exophthalmos ('pop-eye')	- associated with ascites

5. Gill Problems

Symptom	Possible Cause
Pale gills (normal lamellae)	- Anaemia (due to, eg., acute viral and bacterial infections, parasites, nutritional deficiency or toxicity, exogenous toxins).
Pale gills	- Chronic gill damage with (thickened lamellae) epithelial hyperplasia due to, for example, parasites, water quality problems, nutritional gill disease, bacterial gill disease
Excess mucus on gills	- As for skin
Haemorrhages in gills	- Viral infections - infection with *Sanguinicola* sp. - Ectoparasites - Branchiomycosis
White spots on gills	- Ectoparasites (e.g: 'Ich', glochidia, gill maggots)
Marbled and ragged appearance of gills	- Bacterial gill disease - Branchiomycosis

6. General Signs Visible Externally

Symptom	Possible Cause
Ascites and/or 'pop-eye'	- Viral infections - Chronic bacterial disease - exogenous toxins - internal granulomata - internal neoplasia
Translucent faeces	- Gastro-intestinal parasitism resulting in excess mucus production
Trailing faeces	- Constipation
Haemorrhagic faeces	- Intestinal parasitism - acute viral infection - acute bacterial infection
Deformity	- Chronic exposure to some toxins - nutritional toxicity or deficiency

7. Internal Findings

Symptom	Possible Cause
Swellings within muscle	- Tet disease - Parasitic cysts - Granulomata - Neoplasia
Haemorrhagic swimbladder	- Chronic bacterial infection - Swimbladder Inflammation - Myxosporean infestation
White deposits in kidney with 'gritty feel' when cut.	- Nephrocalcinosis
White nodules in gut wall (especially in carp)	- Coccidiosis
Swellings within organs	- Parasitic cysts - Granulomata - Neoplasia
'Worms' free in abdominal cavity	- Intermediate stages of parasites (e.g: *Ligula* sp., *Diphyllobothrium* sp.)
Haemorrhagic gut wall	- Gastro-intestinal parasites - Acute viral disease - Acute bacterial disease
Granulomata	- Old parasitic cysts - Fungal infections - Chronic granulomatous bacterial infections

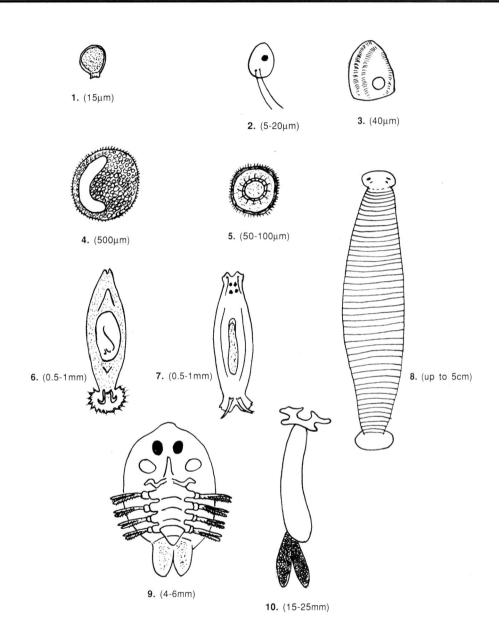

1. (15μm)

2. (5-20μm)

3. (40μm)

4. (500μm)

5. (50-100μm)

6. (0.5-1mm)

7. (0.5-1mm)

8. (up to 5cm)

9. (4-6mm)

10. (15-25mm)

1.	*Oodinium* sp.	**4.**	*Ichthyophthirius* sp.	**7.**	*Dactylogyrus* sp.
2.	*Ichthyobo* sp. (Costia)	**5.**	*Trichodina* sp.	**8.**	Leech
3.	*Chilodonella* sp.	**6.**	*Gyrodactylus* sp.	**9.**	*Argulus* sp.
				10.	*Lernaea* sp.

Adapted from Scott P.W. (1985) in *Manual of Exotic Pets* Revised Edition
(Edited by J.E. Cooper, M.F. Hutchison, O.F. Jackson, R.J. Maurice) B.S.A.V.A. Publications.

1. Weights and Measures

1 cubic metre	:	35.31 cubic feet
1 cubic foot	:	6.22 gallons
		28.3 litres
1 gallon (imp)	:	4.55 litres
1 litre	:	0.22 gallons
1 lb	:	454 grammes
1 Kg	:	2.2 lb
1 mg/litre	:	1 part per million (p.p.m.)
1 ml/1000 litres	:	1 p.p.m.

2. Water Hardness - Comparison of different scales

Scale	Origin	Equiv.in terms of mg/litre $CaCO_3$	Conversion factor to mg/litre $CaCO_3$
°hardness	USA	1 mg/litre $CaCO_3$	-
°Clark	UK	14.3mg/litre $CaCO_3$	14.3
°dH	Germany	17.9mg/litre $CaCO_3$	17.9
°fH	France	20mg/litre $CaCO_3$	20.0

3. Water Hardness - Range of values

Mg/litre $CaCO_3$	°dH	Considered as
0 - 50	3	Soft
50 - 100	3 - 6	Moderately soft
100 - 200	6 - 12	Slightly hard
200 - 300	12 - 18	Moderately hard
300 - 450	18 - 25	Hard
Over 450	Over 25	Very hard

4. Specific gravity / Salinity (at 15°C)

Specific gravity	Salinity (gm/litre)
1.015	20.6
1.016	22.0
1.017	23.3
1.018	24.6
1.019	25.9
1.020	27.2
1.021	28.5
1.022	29.8
1.023	31.1
1.024	32.4
1.025	33.7
Sea Water 1.026	35.0
1.027	36.3
1.028	37.6
1.029	38.9
1.030	40.2

At higher temperatures, the equivalent specific gravity falls.

5. Length/Weight of Fish Conversion

Differences in body shape/conformation make an accurate assessment of a fish's body weight from its length impossible. However, the following figures are a useful "rule of thumb" guide for carp.

Length	Weight
10cm	25g
20cm	115g
30cm	560g

Koi carp are classified into groups according to their colour patterns. These have complex Japanese names, and the reader is referred to standard texts for a complete account.

The following table gives a list of examples

NAME	COLOUR
1. Single colour:	
Shiromuji	White
Benigoi	Red
Hi Matsuba	Red; Pattern of darker scales giving a pine - cone effect
Kigoi	Yellow
2. Metallic colour (Ogon)	
Kin Matsuba	Brown pine - cone pattern on gold.
Parrachina	Platinum - white 'leather'
Gin Matsuba	Platinum with blue pine - cone effect
3. Two colours	
Kohaku	Red on white
Kuchibeni Kohaku	Red lipstick - like pattern
Tancho Kohaku	White with red circle on head
Nidan Kohaku	Two clear patches of red on white
Sandan Kohaku	Three clear patches of red on white
Yondan Kohaku	Four clear patches of red on white
Shiro Bekko	Black on white
Aka Bekko	Black on red
Ki Bekko	Black on yellow
Shiro Utsuri	White on black
Hi Utsuri	Red on black
Ki Utsuri	Yellow on black
Shusui	
Hana Shusui	All Red and blue varieties
Hi Shusui	
4. Three colours	
Taisho Sanke	Red and black on white
Tancho Sanke	As above, although red restricted to circle pattern on head.
Hi Showa	As above, although red predominates and very little white.

5. Scale types

Scaled	Typical scales
Doitsu	Scales along dorsal and lateral lines only
Leather	No visible scales, except possibly very small ones along the dorsal line.
Gin Rin	A gold or silver mirror - like effect on individual scales

REFERENCES AND FURTHER READING

ANATOMY & PHYSIOLOGY

BONE, Q. and MARSHALL, N.B. (1982) *Biology of Fishes.* Blackie, Glasgow.

HARDER, W. (1975) *Anatomy of Fishes* E. Schweitzerbart'sche Verlagsbuchhandlung, Stuttgart.

HOAR, W.S. and RANDALL, D.J. (1969 - present) *Fish Physiology.* Vols I-XI. Academic Press, New York.

LAGLER, K.F., BARDACH, J.E., MILLER, R.R. and PASSINO, D.R.M. (1977). *Ichthylogy. 2nd Edit.* J. Wiley and Sons, New York.

NELSON, J.S. (1984). *Fishes of the World.* 2nd Edit. J. Wiley and Sons, New York.

NILSSON, S. and HOLMGREN, S. (Eds.) (1986) *Fish Physiology : Recent Advances.* Croom Helm, London.

PITCHER, T.J. (Ed.) (1986) *The Behaviour of Teleost Fishes.* Croom Helm, London.

SMITH, L. (1982) *Introduction to Fish Physiology* T.F.H. Publications, New York.

TYTLER, P. and CALOW, P. (Eds.) (1985) *Fish Energetics : New Perspectives.* Croom Helm, London.

WOOTTON, R.J. (1990) *Ecology of Teleost Fishes.* Chapman and Hall, London.

ZUPANC, G.K.H. (1985) *Fish and their Behaviour.* Tetra Press.

NUTRITION

HALVER, J.E. (1972). *Fish Nutrition .* Acedemic Press

JOCHER, W. (1973) . *Live Foods for the Aquarium and Terrarium* T.F.H. Publications, New York (ref No. PS-309)

LOVELL, T. (1989) *Nutrition and Feeding of Fish.* Van Nostrand Reinhard, New York.

MASTERS, C.O. (1975) *Encyclopaedia of Live Foods* T.F.H. Publications, New York. (ref No. PS-730)

STEFFENS, W. (1989) *Principles of Fish Nutrition.* Horwood, Chichester.

GENERAL FISHKEEPING

ADEY, W.H. and LOVELAND, K. (1991) *Dynamic Aquaria.* Academic Press, New York.

ANDREWS, C. (1987). *A Fishkeepers Guide to Fancy Goldfishes* Salamander Books, London

ANDREWS, C., Excell, A. and CARRINGTON, N. (1988). *The Manual of Fish Health.* Salamander Books, London.

BREWSTER, B., CHAPLE, N., CUVELIER, J., DAVIES, M., EVANS, D., EVANS, G., PHIPPS, K. and SCOTT, P.W. (1989). *The Interpet Encyclopedia of Koi.* Salamander Books, London.

CARRINGTON, N. (1985). *A Fishkeeper's Guide to Maintaining a Healthy Aquarium.* Salamander Books, London.

DAWES, J. (1989) *The John Dawes Book of Water Gardens* T.F.H. Publications, New York.

FORD, D.M. (1981) *The Hobby of Ornamental Fishkeeping.* Journal of Small Animal Practice **22** : 317 - 322

JAMES, B. (1986) *A Fishkeepers Guide to Aquarium Plants* Salamander Books, London.

JAMES, B. (1986) *An Interpet Guide to Koi* Salamander Books, London.

MELZAK, M. (1984) *The Marine Aquarium Manual* B.T. Batsford Ltd.

MILLS, D. (1982) *The Practical Encyclopedia of Freshwater Tropical Fishes* Salamander Books, London

MILLS, D. (1987). *The Marine Aquarium.* Salamander Books, London.

MILLS, D., SANDS, D. and SCOTT, P.W. (1988). *A popular guide to Tropical Aquarium Fishes.* Salamander Books, London.

PAPWORTH, D. (1984) *A Fishkeepers Guide to Garden Ponds* Salamander Books, London.

POOLE, T. (Ed) (1987) *The UFAW Handbook on the Care and Management of Laboratory Animals* Longman.

RIEHL R. and BAENSCH H.A. (1987) *Aquarium Atlas* H.A.Baensch Publishers, Melle, Germany.

SCOTT, P.W. (1991). *The Complete Aquarium.* Dorling Kindersley, London.

SPOTTE, S. (1973). *Marine Aquarium Keeping : Science, Animals and Art* Wiley Interscience, New York.

SPOTTE, S. (1979). *Seawater Aquariums: The Captive Environment.* Wiley Interscience, New York.

STERBA, G. (1987). *The Aquarist's Encyclopaedia.* Blandford Press, Poole.

VAN RAMSHORST, J.D. (1978). *The Complete Aquarium Encyclopedia of Tropical Freshwater Fish.* Elsevier-Phaidon, Oxford.

GENERAL PATHOLOGY TEXTS AND BROAD REVIEW ARTICLES

FERGUSON, H. (1989) *Systemic Pathology of Fish* , Iowa State University Press

GRATZEK, J.B. (1981). *An overview of ornamental fish diseases and therapy.* Journal of Small Animal Practice **22**, 345.

HOFFMAN, G.L. and MEYER, F.P. (1974) *Parasites of Freshwater Fishes.* T.F.H. Publications, New York

MAWDESLEY-THOMAS, L.E. (Ed) (1971) *Diseases of Fish* Symposia of the Zoological Soc. of London, Number **30** . Academic Press

POST, G. (1987). *Textbook of Fish Health.* TFH Publications, New York.

RIBELIN, W.E. and MIGAKI, G. (Eds) (1979) *The Pathology of Fishes* The University of Wisconsin Press.

RICHARDS, R.H. (1977) *Diseases of aquarium fish - The Clinical Approach* Vet. Record **101** : 111-113.

RICHARDS, R.H. (1977) *Diseases of aquarium fish - Skin Diseases.* Vet. Record **101** : 132-135.

RICHARDS, R.H. (1977) *Diseases of aquarium fish - Diseases of Internal Organs* Vet. Record **101** : 149-150.

RICHARDS, R.H. (1977) *Diseases of aquarium fish - Treatment* Vet. Record **101** : 166-167.

ROBERTS, R.J. (1989) *Fish Pathology* Bailliere Tindall

SCOTT, P.W. (1981). *Ornamental fishkeeping and the veterinary surgeon* Journal of Small Animal Practice **22** : 331-343

SCOTT, P.W. (1985). Ornamental Fish. In: *Manual of Exotic Pets.* Revised Edition (Eds. J.E. Cooper, M.F. Hutchison, O.F. Jackson, R.J. Maurice). BSAVA Cheltenham.

SCOTT, P.W. (1991). Ornamental Fish. In: *Manual of Exotic Pets.* (Eds. P.H. Beynon and J.E. Cooper) BSAVA Cheltenham.

SNIESZKO, S.F. and AXELROD, H.R. (Eds.) (1970 to 1976). *Diseases of Fishes,* Books 1-5, T.F.H. Publications, New York

STUART, N.C. (1983). *Treatment of fish disease.* Vet. Record **112** : 173-177

VAN DUIJN, C. (1973) *Diseases of Fishes,* 3rd Edition., Iliffe Books, London.

WEBSTER, L.J. (Ed.) (1982). *Aquatic Toxicology* Raven Press, New York.

UNTERGASSER, D. (1989). *Handbook of Fish Diseases.* T.F.H. Publications, Inc. N.J. 07753.

SPECIFIC SUBJECT REFERENCES

ALDERMAN, D.J. (1985). *Malachite green : a review* Journal of Fish Diseases **8** : 289.

ANDREWS, C. and RILEY, A. (1982) *Anthelmintic treatment of fish via stomach tube.* Fisheries Management **13** (2) : 83.

ANON (1989) *Environmental Health Criteria 79. Dichlorvos* International Programme on Chemical Safety. W.H.O.

AUSTIN, B. and AUSTIN, D.A. (1987). *Bacterial Fish Pathogens - Disease in Farmed and Wild Fish.* Ellis Harwood Series. pp 23-42.

BLASIOLA, G.C. (1978) *The use of DTHP.* Aquarist and Pondkeeper (Dec.)

BROWN, L.A. (1981) *Anaesthesia in Fishes.* Journal of Small Animal Practice **22** : 385 - 390.

BROWN, L.A. (1987) *Recirculation anaesthesia for laboratory fish* Laboratory Animals **21** : 210 - 215.

BUTCHER, R.L. and WEARMOUTH, G. (1992) *A survey of health problems in freshly imported tropical fish (Xiphophorus maculatus).* Journal of Small Animal Practice (In Prep).

CARDEILHAC, P.T. and WHITAKER, B.R. (1988). *Copper treatments : Uses and Precautions* In: Tropical Fish Medicine. Veterinary Clinics of North America Small Animal Practice. (Ed. M.K. Stoskopf) **18** (2) : 435. Saunders, Philadelphia.

COOPER, M.E. (1983) *Anaesthesia : The legal requirements* Veterinary Practice 18th April 1983.

COOPER, M.E. (1987). *An introduction to Animal Law* Academic Press, London.

CROSS, D.G. and HURSEY, P.A. (1973) *Chloramine-T for the control of Ichthyophthirius multifiliis (Fouqet).* Journal of Fish Biology. **5** :789.

DEAR, G. (1986). *The use of organophosphorus compounds for the control of fish ectoparasites in ponds.* Institute of Fisheries Management. Nottingham.

DURHAM, P.J.K. and ANDERSON, C.D. (1981). *Lymphocystis disease in imported tropical fish,* N.Z.Vet.J. **29** : 88 - 91.

DOWNING, K. and MERKENS, J. (1955). *The influence of dissolved oxygen concentrations on the toxicity of un-ionised ammonia in rainbow trout (Salmo gairdnerii, Richardson).* Annals of Applied Biology **43** : 243 - 246

EMERSON, K., RUSSO, R.C., LUND, R.E. & THURSTON, R.V. (1975). *Aqueous ammonia equibrium calculations - effect of pH and temperature* Journal Fish Research Bd. Canada **32** : 2379 - 2383.

FRERICHS, G.N. (1984). *The isolation and Identification of Fish Bacterial Pathogens.* Institute of Aquaculture, Stirling, Scotland.

FROMM, P. (1970). *Toxic action of water soluble pollutants on freshwater fishes.* Water Pollution Research Control Series 18050 : 56.

GOVEN, B.A., GILBERT, J.P. and GRATZEK, J.B. (1980) *Apparent drug resistance to the organophosphate dimethyl (2,2,2-trichlor-1-hydroxyethyl) phosphonate by monogenetic trematodes.* Journal of Wildlife Diseases **16** (3): 343.

GOVEN, B.A. and AMEND, D.F. (1980) *Mebendazole/trichlorfon combination : a new anthelmintic for removing monogenetic trematodes from fish.* Journal of Fish Biology **20** (4) : 373.

HERWIG, N. (1979). *Handbook of Drugs and Chemicals used in the Treatment of Fish Diseases : A Manual of Fish Pharmacology and Materia Medica* Charles C. Thomas, Springfield.

HOFFMAN, G.L. and MEYER, F.P. (1974) *Parasites of freshwater fishes. A review of their control and treatment.* T.F.H.Publications, New York.

HOWARTH, W. (1990) *The Law of Aquaculture: The law relating to the farming of fish and shellfish in Britain.* Fishing News Books, Oxford.

HOWARTH, W. (1990) *The Law of the National Rivers Authority.* N.R.A. and Centre for Law in Rural Areas, Aberystwyth.

HYLAND, K. and ADAMS, S. (1987) *Ivermectin for use in fish.* Veterinary Record **120** : 539.

KUDO, S. & KIMURA, N. (1983). *The recovery from hyperplasia in an Artificial Infection.* Bulletin of the Japanese Society of Scientific Fisheries **49** : 1635-1641.

KUDO, S. & KIMURA, N. (1983). *Transmission electron microscopic studies on bacterial gill disease in rainbow trout fingerlings.* Japanese Journal of Ichthyology **30** : 247-260.

LAIRD, L.M. and OSWALD, R.L. (1975). *A note on the use of benzocaine (ethyl p-aminobenzoate) as a fish anaesthetic.* Journal of the Institute of Fisheries Management **6** (4) : 92.

LETEUX, F. and MEYER, F.P. (1972) *Mixtures of malachite green and formalin for controlling Ichthyophthirius and other protozoan parasites of fish.* Progressive Fish Culturist **34** (1) : 21.

LEIBOVITZ, L. (1980). *Lymphocystis Disease,* J.A.V.M.A. **176** : 202.

LEIBOVITZ, L. (1980). *Ichthyophthirius* J.A.V.M.A. **176** : 30 - 31.

LEIBOVITZ, L. (1980). *Fish Tuberculosis (mycobacteriosis)*, J.A.V.M.A. **176** : 415.

LEIBOVITZ, L., RIIS, R.C. and GEORGI, M.E. (1980). *Diseases of aquarium fish : Digenetic trematode infection* . J.A.V.M.A. **177** : 40 - 42.

LEIBOVITZ, L. and PINELLO, C. (1980). *Mycotic infections* J.A.V.M.A. **177** : 1110 - 1112.

LEIBOVITZ, L. (1980). *Fish Tuberculosis (mycobacteriosis)*, J.A.V.M.A. **176** : 415.

McFARLAND, W.N. (1960) *The use of anesthetics for the handling and the transport of fishes* Calif. Fish Game **46** : 407 -431

MULERTT, H. (1902) *The goldfish and its systematic culture.* 3rd Edition, Brooklyn.

OBERMEIER, P. (1974) *Modern drugs for fish. Masoten: Ectoparasite control.* Veterinary Medical Review **2** : 172.

O'GRADY, P., PALMER, R., HICKEY, C. and SMITH, P.R. (1986) *Antibiotic therapy of furunculosis in freshwater and seawater* In: Pathology in Marine Aquaculture. (Eds. C.P. Vivares, J.R. Bonami and E. Jaspers). European Mariculture Society. Special Bulletin No.9. Bredene, Belgium.

PESUT, A.P., and GOLDSCHMIDT, M. (1983). *Selected Integumentary Diseases of Tropical Freshwater Fish.* The Compendium on Continuing Education **5** : 343-358.

POOL, D., RYDER, K. and ANDREWS, C. (1984) *The control of Bothriocephalus acheilognathi in Grass Carp, Ctenopharyngodon idella, using praziquantel.* Fisheries Management **15** (1) : 31.

POST, G. (1971). *Systematic Grading of gill hyperplasia.* Progress Fish Culture **33** : 61.

RIJKERS, G.T., TEUNISSEN, A.G., VAN OOSTEROM, R. and VAN MUISWINKEL, W.B. (1980) *The immune system of cyprinid fish. The immunosuppressive effect of the antibiotic oxytetracycline in carp. (Cyprinus carpio).* Aquaculture **19** :177-189.

RUSSO, R.C., THURSTON, R.V., and EMERSON, K. (1981). *Acute toxicity of nitrite to rainbow trout (Salmo gairdnerii) : Effects of pH nitrate species and anion species.* Can. Journal Fish. Aquat. Sci. **38** : 387 - 393.

SCOTT, P.W. and FOGLE, B. (1983) *Treatment of koi carp (Cyprinus carpio L) infected with anchor worms (Lernaea cyprinacea L).* Veterinary Record **113** (18) : 421.

SCOTT, P.W. (1982) *Chemical disease control.* Fish Farmer **5** (6) : 35.

SCOTT, P.W. (1983) *Fish farm checklist.* Veterinary Record **112** (9) : 198-200.

SNIESZKO, S.F. (1974) *The effects of environmental stress on outbreaks of infectous diseases of fish.* Journal of Fish Biology **6** : 197 - 208.

SHOTTS, E.B., KLECHNER, A.C., GRATZEK, J.B. & BLUE, J.C. (1976). *Bacterial Flora of Aquarium Fishes and their Shipping Waters Imported from South East Asia.* Journal Fish Research Bd. Canada **33** : 732 - 735.

SOMMERVILLE, C. (1981) *Parasites of ornamental fish* Journal of Small Animal Practice **22** :367 - 376.

STOSKOPF, M.K. (1988) *Fish Chemotherapeutics.* In: Tropical Fish Medicine. Veterinary Clinics of North America Small Animal Practice. (Ed. M.K. Stoskopf.) **18** (2) : 329.

STOSKOPF, M.K. (1990) *Shark diagnostics and therapeutics: a short review.* Journal of Aquariculture and Aquatic Science **5** (3) : 33.

STUART, N.C. (1979) *A critical review of the literature on the anaesthesia of fishes* M.Sc. Thesis. University of Stirling.

STUART, N.C. (1981) *Anaesthetics in Fishes* Journal of Small Animal Practice **22** :377 - 384.

STUART, N.C. (1983) *Treatment of fish disease.* Veterinary Record **112** :173-177

STUART, N.C. (1988). *Common skin diseases of farmed and pet fish* In Practice **10** :47-53.

THURSTON, R.V., RUSSO, R.C. and SMITH, C.E. (1978). *Acute toxicity of ammonia and nitrite to cutthroat trout fry.* Trans. Am. Fish. Soc. **107** : 361 - 365

VAN DUIJN, C. (1981). *Tuberculosis on Fishes.* Journal of Small Animal Practice **22** : 391.

WOOD, E.M. and JOHNSON, H.E. (1957) *Acute sulphamethazine toxicity in young salmon.* Progressive Fish Culturist **19** : 64.

YATES, R. (1955) *A new treatment for finrot and fungus* Aquarist and Pondkeeper , September 1955.

JOURNALS AND MAGAZINES

Annual Review of Fish Diseases Pergamon Press, Oxford
Aquatic Sciences and Fisheries Abstracts FAO., Rome.

Journal of Fish Biology Academic Press, London
Journal of Fish Diseases (Edited by R.J. Roberts) Blackwell Scientific Publications

The Aquarist and Pondkeeper Published by Dog World, 9 Tufton Street, Ashford, Kent.
Practical Fishkeeping Published by EMAP Pursuit Publications Ltd., Bretton Court, Bretton, Peterborough, PE3 8DZ.

USEFUL ADDRESSES

Aquarian Advisory Service, P.O. Box 67, Elland, West Yorkshire HX5 0S.

Institute of Aquaculture, University of Stirling, Stirling, Scotland FK9 4LA.

MAFF - Weymouth Fisheries Laboratory, The Lookout House, The Nothe, Weymouth, Dorset DT4 8UB.

Ornamental Fish International, Keith Baraclough Aquarist Ltd, Hayfield Mills, Haycliffe Lane, Bradford, West Yorkshire BD5 9ET.

INDEX

LIST OF B.S.A.V.A. PUBLICATIONS

THE JOURNAL OF SMALL ANIMAL PRACTICE

An International Journal Published Monthly   Editor W. D. Tavernor, B.V.Sc., PhD., F.R.C.V.S.
Fifteen Year Cumulative Index published 1976
Available by post from: B.S.A.V.A. Administration Office, Kingsley House, Church Lane,
Shurdington, Cheltenham, Gloucestershire GL51 5TQ

Manual of Parrots, Budgerigars and other Psittacine Birds
Edited by C.J. Price, M.A., Vet. M.B., M.R.C.V.S.
B.S.A.V.A. Publications Committee 1988

Manual of Laboratory Techniques
New Edition
Edited by D.L. Doxey, B.V.M. & S., Ph.D., M.R.C.V.S.
and M. B. F. Nathan, M.A., B.V.Sc., M.R.C.V.S.
B.S.A.V.A. Publications Committee 1989

Manual of Anaesthesia for Small Animal Practice
Third Revised Edition
Edited by A. D. R. Hilbery, B.Vet., Med., M.R.C.V.S.
B.S.A.V.A. Publications Committee 1992

Manual of Radiography and Radiology in Small Animal Practice
Edited by R. Lee, B.V.Sc., D.V.R., Ph D., M.R.C.V.S.
B.S.A.V.A. Publications Committee 1989

Manual of Small Animal Neurology
Edited by S.J. Wheeler, B.V.Sc, Cert, V.R., Ph.D., M.R.C.V.S.
B.S.A.V.A. Publications Committee 1989

Manual of Small Animal Dentistry
Edited by C.E. Harvey, B.V.Sc., F.R.C.V.S., Dip.A.C.V.S., Dip.A.V.D.C.
and H. S. Orr, B.V.Sc., M.R.C.V.S., D.V.R.
B.S.A.V.A. Publications Committee 1990

Manual of Small Animal Endocrinology
Edited by M.F. Hutchison, B.Sc., B.V.M.S., M.R.C.V.S.
B.S.A.V.A. Publications Committee 1990

Manual of Exotic Pets
New Edition
Edited by P.H. Beynon, B.V.Sc., M.R.C.V.S.
and J.E. Cooper, B.V.Sc., Cert. L.A.S., D.T.V.M., F.R.C.V.S., M.C.R. Path., F.I. Biol.
B.S.A.V.A. Publications Committee 1991

Manual of Small Animal Oncology
Edited by
R.A.S. White, B.Vet.Med., PhD., D.V.R., F.R.C.V.S.,
Diplomate, American College of Veterinary Surgeons
B.S.A.V.A. Publications Committee 1991

Manual of Canine Behaviour
Second Edition
Valerie O'Farrell, Ph.D., Chartered Psychologist
B.S.A.V.A. Publications Committee 1992

Manual of Ornamental Fish
Edited by R. L. Butcher, M.A., Vet.M.B., M.R.C.V.S.
B.S.A.V.A. Publications Committee 1992

Manual of Reptiles
Editor by P.H. Beynon, B.V.Sc., M.R.C.V.S.,
J. E. Cooper, B.V.Sc., Cert. L.A.S. , D.T.V.M., F.R.C.V.S., M.C.R. Path., F.I. Biol.
and M.P.C. Lawton, B.Vet.Med., Cert.V. Ophthal., F.R.C.V.S.
B.S.A.V.A. Publications Committee 1992

B.S.A.V.A. VIDEO 1 (VHS and BETA)
Radiography and Radiology of the Canine Chest
Presented by R. Lee, B.V.Sc., D.V.R., Ph.D., M.R.C.V.S.
Edited by M. McDonald, B.V.M.S., M.R.C.V.S.
B.S.A.V.A. Publications Committee 1983

An introduction to Veterinary Anatomy and Physiology
By A. R. Michell, B.Vet.Med., Ph.D., M.R.C.V.S.
and P.E. Watkins, M.A., Vet.M.B., M.R.C.V.S., D.V.R.
B.S.A.V.A. Publications Committee 1989

Proceedings of the B.S.A.V.A. Symposium "Improved Healthcare in Kennels and Catteries"
Edited by P.H. Beynon, B.V.Sc., M.R.C.V.S.
B.S.A.V.A. Publications Committee 1991

Practical Veterinary Nursing
Second Revised Edition
Edited by C.J. Price, M.A., Vet.M.B., M.R.C.V.S.
B.S.A.V.A. Publications Committee 1991

Practice Resource Manual
Edited by D.A. Thomas, B.Vet.Med., M.R.C.V.S.
B.S.A.V.A. Publications Committee 1992

AVAILABLE FROM BOOKSELLERS

Canine Medicine and Therapeutics
Third Edition
Edited by E.A. Chandler, B.Vet.Med., F.R.C.V.S.,
D.J. Thompson, B.A., M.V.B., M.R.C.V.S.,
J.B. Sutton, M.R.C.V.S.
and C.J. Price, M.A., Vet.M.B., M.R.C.V.S.
Blackwell Scientific Publications 1991.

An Atlas of Canine Surgical Techniques
Edited by P.G.C. Bedford, Ph.D., B.Vet. Med., F.R.C.V.S., D.V. Ophthal.
Blackwell Scientific Publications 1984

Feline Medicine and Therapeutics
Edited by E.A. Chandler, B.Vet.Med., F.R.C.V.S.,
C.J. Gaskell, B.V.Sc., Ph.D., D.V.R., M.R.C.V.S.
and A.D.R. Hilbery, B.Vet.Med., M.R.C.V.S.
Blackwell Scientific Publications 1985

Jones's Animal Nursing
Fifth Edition
Edited by D.R. Lane, B.Sc., F.R.C.V.S.
Pergamon Press 1989